Healing 101

A guide to creating the foundation
for complete wellness

By Theresa Ramsey, N.M.D.

Center for Natural Healing Press

Healing 101
Copyright © 2006 Theresa Ramsey, N.M.D.
Center for Natural Healing Press

All rights reserved. No part of this book may be reproduced (except for inclusion in reviews), disseminated or utilized in any form or by any means, electronic or mechanical, including photocopying, recording, or in any information storage and retrieval system, or the Internet/World Wide Web without written permission from the author or publisher.

For more information about this title, please contact:
Center for Natural Healing Press
9015 E. Via Linda, Suite 107-313
Scottsdale, Arizona 85258
E-mail: healing101@healthhappens.net

Book design by:
Arbor Books
www.arborbooks.com

Printed in United States

Theresa Ramsey, N.M.D.
Healing 101

Library of Congress Control Number: 2005906653
ISBN: 0-9771512-0-4

I dedicate this book to my children—for without you both, it would not have been possible. You two boys teach me more about life than anyone else. You bring me home to my heart—always. Bless you.

Acknowledgements

Without question, this book would not have been written without the countless number of patients who willingly chose to invest in their healing process—their time, their money, their courage and persistence. So, for you my patients, your support and belief in me are among the biggest blessings in my life. You have all made an impact on the history of a changing medicine—one that is essential for the necessary shift of our planet towards healing and love rather than illness, fear and fighting. Thank you for hearing that healing doesn't have to be a fight and for recognizing that your personal healing goes beyond physical health. A special thank you to each patient who has been with me from the very beginning—at times it was simply your faith in me that kept me going.

Thank you also to the beginning class of Southwest College of Naturopathic Medicine—we were the pioneers and had the best of the best as the school began its history. Thank you to the many teachers who flew in from around the country and the world to guide each of us with your individual artistic healing gifts. You gave us the courage and belief to commit to providing a controversial and not so well accepted form of medicine to those seeking this type of knowledge. I'd like to acknowledge the students of SCNM for allowing me to remind you that healing is an art, an individual journey and expression of the self.

A special thank you to my family for tolerating the time I have spent with this project—this newest member of our family as it truly felt like birthing all over again, not just for me but for each of us as a family. We can look back now and realize that times like these bring us closer, although it doesn't feel that way at the time. Your support and belief in me mean more to me than words can explain. And to you, Mom and Dad, thank you for having the courage to allow me to live my life just a little bit differently than most people. You've supported me even when you didn't know how to and this has certainly not gone unnoticed. We've all grown together and for all of you I am grateful.

I'd like to thank each reader in advance for having the wisdom to know that there is much more to this lifetime than what most of us are told. You are already a part of the solution to this ever-changing world.

Contents

Introduction 1

Part I

Medicine and Healing

Chapter 1—Wellness-Illness Continuum 5
Chapter 2—Reconnecting to the Missing Piece 16
Chapter 3—Insurance ≠ Assurance 19
Chapter 4—How It Has Been Is Not How It Is 25
Chapter 5—One Step At A Time 27
Chapter 6—The One-on-One Experience. 33
Chapter 7—The Naturopathic Medical Approach. 36
Chapter 8—Difficult but Simple. 38
　　　　　　　Inventory Time 42
Chapter 9—A Chronic Problem 43
Chapter 10—Evolution. 47
Chapter 11—Where Do You Fit?. 51

Part II

The Mind

Chapter 12—Healing the Mind-Body Relationship. . . . 53
　　　　　　　　Notice Your Story. 58
　　　　　　　　Example of Noticing My Story. 59
Chapter 13—Learning to Love. 60
　　　　　　　　Feel Your Story 67
Chapter 14—Choosing Love 68
　　　　　　　　Change Your Story. 76
　　　　　　　　The New You 77

Part III

The Body

Chapter 15—Coming Home 78
          Your Body in Your Life 82
Chapter 16—Nurture Yourself 83
          Weekly Food Planner 94
Chapter 17—Letting Go 95
          Keys to Enhance Elimination 101
Chapter 18—Movement 102
Chapter 19—Your Shock Absorbers 105
          Pause and Breathe 110
Chapter 20—Relationships. 111
          Mirror, Mirror on the Wall. 114

Part IV

The Spirit

Chapter 21—Surrender 115
          Turning the Fragmented You
          into the Integrated You 119
Chapter 22—Gratitude. 120
          The Gratitude Journal 126
Chapter 23—Forgiveness 127
Chapter 24—Love 130

Part V

Healing Paths

Chapter 25—Same Condition, Different Journey 134
Chapter 26—The Real Deal 144

Naturopathic Organizations 147
Naturopathic Medical Schools .148
Commonly Asked Questions 150

Healing 101

Introduction

As a naturopathic physician, I witness illness and healing in ways that I wasn't prepared for emotionally or intellectually in medical school. I realize that the reason the practice of medicine is called "practice" is because each and every day I am continuing to learn how to facilitate healing. My patients teach me things that the medical books don't even touch upon.

Accidents to me are "acts of dents" . . . bumps in the road that shape us into who we are today. Each purposely occurs uniquely for our growth. If we allow ourselves the opportunity to be grateful for the dent that slowed us down and got our attention—that knock on the door that asks if we're paying attention—we can receive the full gift of the "accident."

I was certain that becoming a student of the Naturopathic School was a big accident; quarter after quarter, I wanted to drop out. The language, the philosophy—none of it made sense. My language for the previous ten years was of surgery, intensive care and emergency rooms. Now, I was in school learning about the vibration of herbs and the energy lines that ran through our body and about shaved carrots for sore throats and pieces of potato for hemorrhoids. All of this was very entertaining and fun, but it wasn't until I started clinic rotations and witnessed healing in ways I could never before even imagine that I realized my perseverance was completely and totally worth it.

I did, however experience a "BIG ACCIDENT" that changed my life as a physician forever. So here I was—this absolutely nerdy, front-row student who was always at least ten minutes early with all the possible books that might be used, sitting attentively and waiting anxiously for the next bizarre instructor to come and entertain me with facts I was sure I'd never hear anywhere else in the entire world. A much-respected teacher who had published several books and was world-renowned for his work stood in front of me, lecturing on endometriosis. This is a condition in women where the blood that is formed in the uterus backs up into the pelvic cavity, causing severe discomfort. "She was bleeding from her vagina and she was bleeding from her navel and she was bleeding from her eyes . . ." (He said the word "bleeeeeeeeeding" as though it had ten "e's" in it.) Out of nowhere came my voice: "Oh, come on!" It was very out of character for me to be so rude and impulsive. The room was silent. He stood up, leaned over the podium and said, "Young lady, only the wise aren't surprised." He very gently went back to his lecture and I, very angry and embarrassed, proceeded to write his words down on a piece of paper, not knowing a thing about what they meant.

That accidental outburst that spewed out of my mouth that day has affected me as a physician more than any other single event that occurred during medical school. I received the gift of non-judgment. It is clear to me now that if I ever judge one thing a patient brings to my office, at that very moment, I stop assisting them and I stop growing as a physician and as a person—I forfeit my responsibility. How can I participate in the intimate act of healing if I judge what they are saying?

Judgment is a form of resistance. It is a clear, unmistakable emotion. Resistance isn't only felt in the mind and in the heart—it produces a real sensation in the body. The feeling is one that opposes harmony and completeness. I have learned from my patients that the most important gift a patient can receive in going to a health care practitioner is to be accepted and to be heard—accepted for their strengths and weaknesses equally, with their goals and desires being understood. If a physician, in any way, judges what a patient brings to the visit, he is not in harmony within himself, let alone with the person being treated. If, on the other hand, the physician accepts the patient's story completely, he can truly understand what the patient is asking for. The moment judgment surfaces, the resistance puts a barrier between the physician and the patient, and the healing process stops.

I recognize that it takes more wisdom than knowledge to be an effective healer. A philosopher once said, "Knowledge is of the past, wisdom is of the future." There is much truth to this. Healing occurs from today forward. The past is what has made you who you are today. Today makes you who you will be tomorrow. It is necessary for us to begin breaking the binary patterns of right and wrong, always and never, better and worse—as these judgments make us resist our full potential to be complete, integrated, harmonious, healthy, and free beings.

Only the wise aren't surprised. I invite you to breathe and to be open to all possibilities. Your body and your world are depending on you.

∞ Chapter 1 ∞

Medicine and Healing

∫

Wellness-Illness Continuum

This book was inspired by the numerous times I've been asked the same question—"What is Naturopathic Medicine?" I realized that the answer wasn't simple *and* that the answer would vary depending upon who you asked. My definition today is much different than what it was when I was in medical school.

My definition of Naturopathic Medicine today has matured significantly from when I first learned of the field of naturopathy while practicing as a nurse in conventional medicine. Conventional medicine is also known as allopathic medicine. Allopathic physicians are conventional medical physicians, as opposed to Naturopathic physicians, who have a foundation in naturopathy. Naturopathy is a system of therapeutics in which neither medicinal agents nor surgery is used. Naturopathic Medicine has evolved from naturopathy into a licensed and regulated field of medicine. Naturopathic Medical Doctors are primary care physicians who are trained in and licensed to practice naturopathy in addition to prescribing medications and performing minor surgery. There exist unlicensed naturopaths who have studied herbology, homeopathy and nutrition but haven't completed premed requirements for a licensed medical school where training in physical and clinical diagnosis, along with study of pathology, takes place, nor do they sit for board exams. In essence, they are not doctors of medicine, and cannot diagnose and treat disease. The term Naturopathic Medical Doctor and Naturopathic Physician are used interchangeably for licensed primary care physicians who emphasize naturopathic therapeutics.

Coming from my many years of being immersed in allopathic medicine as a nurse, I found myself as a student both inspired and overwhelmed with the field of naturopathy. There appeared to be an endless list of possibilities to choose from to treat all of the ailments that conventional medicine treats with drugs and surgery. Natural therapeutics consist of herbs, nutrients, homeopathic remedies, acupuncture points, dietary practices and exercises not just for physical strength but to enhance breathing, to strengthen eyesight, to facilitate digestion, to align the focus of thought processes, and so forth. All of the limitless possibilities, from dietary changes to mind-body medicine, could be used to address the same condition! The overwhelming variety of treatment options made me appreciate my life as a nurse, where the practice was focused and straightforward. In the allopathic world, guidelines are established with algorithms to follow for the condition being treated. Due to the ease and simplicity of nursing, I frequently pondered the possibility of dropping out of Naturopathic Medical School.

"Standards of care" are what created algorithmic medicine, which is a flow chart with the condition at the top and arrows and boxes guiding you through the best choices to make based on symptoms and responses by the patient. The work was done, medicine became standardized, and all I had to do was follow the chart. My life experiences told me that these particular standards of care, although reproducible, were not where my experience as a health care practitioner was going to end.

Being a nurse, I had a lot of friends who were nurses. Some of the doctors with whom I worked closely also became friends. This was my network, my social group. At the time, I was a vegetarian, I exercised routinely in addition to riding my bicycle to work, and I enjoyed excellent physical health. I remember daily being teased by my friends and peers about the tofu I'd bring to lunch or the helmet I kept in my locker or the yoga postures I could get twisted into. By living life as I felt comfortable, I began to realize what a tremendous source of inadvertent entertainment I offered my friends. So, here we are in the operating room, talking together over an open chest while we sewed a new vessel to someone's dying heart, and I'm being teased about *my* quirky lifestyle!

I laughed along with everybody else, as it did seem funny that nobody else in that room chose to live as I did.

We all got along so well that I didn't notice our differences, or, for that matter, even care about them. I truly loved every minute I was in surgery. The human body is fascinating to explore. Surgery itself is a phenomenal experience, with the many wondrous possible ways to fix people with knives, saws, thread, staples, and artificial pieces to implant! Not a day passed that I didn't look forward to going to work.

But then I started to think about which surgeon I would have perform my open heart surgery if I ever needed it. It was hard for me to fathom the idea of anyone being the right one, although I respected them all very much. I just couldn't plan the possibility. This opened the door for me to realize that I was creating, more at a subconscious level than otherwise, the least likely outcome for me, which would be open heart surgery. I was preventing unwanted outcomes. If, one day, it becomes my destiny to require surgical assistance with my heart—I'll be able to make the best choice for me then. This marked the beginning of opening my awareness to health in a new way.

We were back in the operating room enjoying light conversation about the tofu stir fry I made the night before and my date to hike Camelback Mountain afterwards. Laughter is always helpful in the operating room. Now, I was really starting to think about the quirkiness of sawing a chest open in order to get to our patient's failing heart. We got into his chest and purposely created a flat line on the EKG. We did this by shunting all of the patient's blood away from the heart using a machine to pump his blood so the heart could be still while we created new plumbing. In the process, we moved his anatomy around by bringing a vessel from his leg to his heart. I don't know about you, but, to me, this started to seem quirkier than eating well and staying active!

Open heart surgery has saved many lives and will continue to do so. My intention is not to belittle the procedure. I share this story to give you my perspective on myself as I chose this role in medicine while, at the same time living a vigorous life that gave me great joy simply because I felt good in the moment. At the time, my decisions weren't based on preventing a future heart attack. My actions were natural for who I was. All of a sudden I started looking at the role I was choosing as a health care provider, and felt that my efforts might be better served in a different arena.

This is why, even though naturopathy appeared so complex while lacking standards of care, I continued my strenuous study of Naturopathic Medicine. As a nurse I was becoming uninspired treating conditions; instead, I wanted to treat people. I was intrigued by all of the talk of wellness and prevention. I had never been surrounded by so many people who shared the same ideas about health and disease. I was beginning to feel as though conventional medicine provided "illness doctors" and I was studying to become a "wellness doctor." This mere definition provided my study with so much joy!

As a student, I was surprised to hear case after case of how therapies other than medications and surgery treated conditions. It was a whole new language and seemed completely worth all of my effort, time and money.

I often worried about how on earth I would know how to choose an herb from the Native American culture or from Eastern Indian Ayurvedic culture or to use a traditional Chinese formula, as they all have biochemical properties appropriate to treat the condition at hand. Each new herb brought me more delight in the possibilities of therapies for my future patients while at the same time bringing me more confusion. I just chose, for survival's sake, to stay focused on what I was being presented with in each class.

When it came to my nutritional training, I found it to be not only inspiring, but also rather surprising, as I was never introduced to the study of how nutrition affected our biochemistry before, even though I had been a nurse for ten years! This opened a whole new way of appreciating the body. As I began learning to apply nutritional supplementation to fill the gaps created by nutritional deficiencies, my image of the body came alive! Biochemistry had previously never been very interesting to me except insofar as I had to pass the tests. Biochemistry with the understanding of nutrient influence and manipulation of our overall health was a whole other ballgame. It became one of my most passionate studies.

During my training, my definition of Naturopathic Medicine at the time would have been *using natural remedies such as supplements, herbs and homeopathy along with nutritional counseling to heal the body*. I realize now that this definition is why the field of Naturopathic Medicine isn't more commonplace. I understand why conventional doctors, or "real doctors," as my patients refer to them, don't readily accept Naturopathic Medicine as a valuable form of medicine. I understand why some insurance companies haven't provided funding for Naturopathic Medical Doctors.

A single herb or a single change in dietary practices can certainly provide better experiences and very well may be the reason someone gets interested in natural healing, but it absolutely does not capture a glimmer of the essence of the field of Naturopathic Medicine. If we are simply replacing a drug with an herb, it isn't a different practice; it is the same, just with an expanded Physician's Desk Reference (PDR). The PDR describes the full scope of a drug to be used for identifiable conditions. We can do this with herbs and nutrients just the same as we do with drugs. There are plenty of books already available that are references for just this.

The past nine years of clinical practice has taught me that Naturopathic Medicine is much richer than choosing healing modalities distinct from surgery and medications. It is true that we do laboratory testing and write prescriptions for X-rays and medications and make referrals to other physicians. We communicate with insurance companies through ICD-9 codes and CPT codes. We do it all, including pap smears and minor surgery.

The difference is in our approach to the wellness-illness continuum. My naturopathic training gave me an appreciation of the many facets that contribute to a person's ease or dis-ease. Drugs and herbs are great tools, but the important question is *how did this person get to this level of health or illness*?

Rather than jumping to the pathology and starting there by cutting it out or suppressing it, I start by listening to things that may have contributed to the path of lack-of-ease or resistance in the patient's biochemistry or physiology somewhere. If there is no resistance, there is ease. If there is ease, there is lack of disease.

This is why, although herbs and supplements have wonderfully unique properties and influence our biochemistry in very specific ways, they do not have the same effect on patient after patient. Ever so frequently I hear a patient tell me that they tried this or that and it didn't work. This is because they were practicing naturopathy, not Naturopathic Medicine.

As people, we are individually complex, starting from the composition of our unique genetic coding, to our choices, to our exposures, to our beliefs, desires, and values. This brings up the physical body's interplay with the mind and the spirit. All of these factors create our unique vibrational frequency, which flows into and out of and around each visible cell, creating the unseen vastness which is the home of our own true self. With the complex uniqueness of each of us, many things create our health or lack of it. Similarly, our physiology is not a singular, unidirectional experience. A single step in the behavior of our physiology is influenced by pathways that are both feeding and receiving information from that step, which itself is influenced by the millions of possible other pathways contributing to it! Our cells communicate to each other in numerous, multiple, absolutely mind-boggling ways! Due to this vast ever-exchanging physiology, the body can fail to benefit from a single tool from nature, although that tool may seemingly be the answer.

Although medicine has provided miraculous cures for acute illnesses or acute outcomes of chronic conditions, chronic illnesses and conditions that may not yet have manifested their acute outcome deserve much more respect and exploration than the medical field is able to give them today.

Conventional medicine lacks the time and training to appropriately address these chronic situations. It is simply not feasible to expect conventional medicine to perform this role. We must be fair in our expectations. At the same time, we must be active in opening the awareness of those who haven't had the privilege to know that there is a kind of medicine that does address these issues—just not where they are used to looking. The very purpose of this book is to do just that—to communicate to the world that Naturopathic Medicine is a viable, growing field that is unique in its ability to prevent future illnesses and to heal chronic illnesses. Due to the unique approach that Naturopathic Medical Doctors use in the healing process, it cannot be compared to conventional medicine as an orange is to an orange. It is an apple to an orange comparison, both necessary and valuable.

Naturopathic Medicine is the body of medicine that respects the unique complexity of each individual, honoring the fact that many potential healing tools can contribute to the healing experience. The healing experience is reflected in the harmony that an individual is able to create with tools of the "physical body," "mind body" and "spirit body."

Neither I nor anyone I know is the expert on understanding which path or therapeutic plan will be THE answer for any one person. Just because I respect our individual rarity or exclusiveness does not mean that I have the grand healing tool that could make you better. Naturopathic Healing is truly a journey for both the patient and the doctor. We are all unique, not only in our physical health, but in the path we chose leading to the creation of who we are today.

This book is designed to help you understand how to bring the power of healing into your life. The purpose of this book is to help you create an energetic and physical space within you to allow whatever tool you choose to assist your healing—whether it's an herb, a nutrient, a medication or a surgery—to have its desired effect.

Each part of this book is an extension of or a complement to the others. You will notice that I continually refer to *ease* vs. *lack-of-ease* or *dis-ease*. This is the wellness-illness continuum. The commonality is whether or not ease is present in the person's experience. It's that simple.

On the surface it appears easy but it takes active, committed, conscious awareness. This book has woven through it exercises designed to bring you closer to recognizing ease or lack of it in your life. The reason this practice is not more commonplace is because not many of our teachers taught us this way of living—hence the epidemic of chronic disease. Whether or not you know about the health of people in your life, look around you and notice if you see a chronic "lack-of-ease" in their existence. Are your friends, coworkers and family members happy and joyful and full of positive things to say and to share—or not?

This book is about reconnecting to the self and to your own guidance system, which will influence your personal internal health as well as your external health. External health is the ease that you experience in your relationships, with your children and extended family, with your coworkers, in your home, and in your finances. This book is designed to help you recognize the true quality of your life. It offers you tools to enhance your life experience, which is a reflection of your internal health and vice-versa. This book helps you to see what your tendencies and patterns have been. Although they may seem natural to you, they may not be natural to your healing process. In summary, this book is about your true nature—love and joy.

In addition, my hope is that this book will be the beginning of a complementary bridge between conventional and naturopathic medicine. I have personally witnessed players from both fields judging or acting as if there is not a need for the other. Not only is this unfortunate for the physicians themselves, this is a tremendous misfortune for the patient who tries to do the best for himself but has physicians that are opposing one another, leaving the patient unsupported. I do believe that if an herb can replace a drug in an equally effective manner that the gentler choice should be made, of course. Healing is about honor, recognizing when a gentle influence such as a nutrient or homeopathic remedy could assist healing, while also being able to know when surrendering to the necessity of a drug or surgery is essential.

Healing is meant to be a joyful experience. Healing is a much more natural state than being sick. As you heal, fewer and fewer tools are needed because you will access the power within you to be one—one complete, vibrant, joyful and healthy being.

∞ *Chapter 2* ∞

Medicine and Healing

∫

Reconnecting to the Missing Piece

One of my favorite authors of children's books is Shel Silverstein. His first book, *The Missing Piece*, inspires people through its simplicity. It's a clear message to all of us that we tend to look outside of ourselves for answers that already exist in complete form within ourselves.

In the same way, medicine plays a very powerful position in society. We surrender our power to it when we are vulnerable. When our health suffers on some level, we turn to the medical field for help. We are extremely fortunate to have this system of medicine. Conventional medicine is fabulous at treating emergencies and acute situations that need immediate attention. This is what conventional doctors are trained to do and this is what insurance pays for—an efficient system that has worked for hundreds of years.

But what about the ailments that medicine hasn't helped us with, like weight management, fatigue, and chronic pain (such as in fibromyalgia or arthritis)? And what about the questions specifically addressing the aging process? There are way too many memory problems, fatigue, aches, and pains as we age. What about the chronic headaches and premenstrual symptoms contributing to days off work, not to mention days off your life? And, are you even aware of underlying conditions existing silently today, that one day can manifest, out of the blue, into an acute symptom that appeared to just surface that day? *Surface* is the correct term, as all acute symptoms have been brewing for some time. Nothing just occurs in the moment that it appears.

What happens when we go to our doctors for these chronic conditions? How would your doctor guide you if you asked for assistance in preventing family-linked illnesses? A recent patient shared with me a comment that his doctor made in response to his complaint of daily knee aches—"Welcome to middle age." Similarly, a forty-three year old, a very fit and actively competitive athlete, was told by his doctor that his knee pain was just part of the game of getting old.

If you've ever been placed on a drug to lower your cholesterol, think back to whether or not your doctor first mentioned how diet, exercise and stress affect your cholesterol and cardiac health. I once had a patient who was thirty-five years old and placed on a medication to lower his blood pressure. As a result of the medication, his blood pressure came down nicely but he became extremely fatigued. He was 5'9" and weighed 357 pounds. When he came to me I did not stop his medication initially; I began working with diet and exercise. He lost 80 pounds and his blood pressure became very low. When he came off of his medication, his energy level immediately improved. I found out a few weeks later that his most recent claim for insurance coverage for my treatment of his hypertension was denied *because* I was treating obesity first, which obviously was the cause of his high blood pressure but which was considered to be much more cost-consuming than treating hypertension.

So, as you read the above examples, I ask you to ponder. . .what is health care all about and why do we fear not having health insurance?

∞ Chapter 3 ∞

Medicine and Healing

$$\int$$

Insurance ≠ Assurance

For the most part, insurance companies fear covering chronic conditions. Is this because medicine hasn't effectively handled these physical conditions? If there were an effective treatment ("effective" means "cost-effective" in this instance), insurance would consider paying for it, right? The number of people afflicted with chronic health complaints is astronomical. Chronic conditions that disturb our quality of life are, unfortunately, an epidemic in our society.

Consider these facts provided by The National Center for Disease Control and Prevention (CDC). All of the information below has come directly from the CDC website.

- Chronic diseases—such as heart disease, cancer, and diabetes—are the leading causes of death and disability in the United States, accounting for 7 out of every 10 deaths and affecting the quality of life of 90 million Americans.

- Obesity has risen at an epidemic rate during the past twenty years in the United States, and has reached epidemic proportions. 65% of U.S. adults are either overweight or obese. Among children, 16% of those between 6 and 19 years old are overweight.

- Diabetes in adults has increased substantially over the past decade—70% among 30-39-year-olds, 40% percent among 40-49-year-olds, and 31% among 50-59-year olds.

- One of every four U.S. deaths is due to cancer. Over 1.3 million new cases will be diagnosed in 2005.

- Poor diet and physical inactivity lead to 300,000 deaths each year—second only to tobacco use.

- People who are overweight or obese increase their risk of cardiovascular disease, diabetes and high blood pressure, arthritis-related disabilities and some cancers.

The medicine that we invest in reflects the needs of today, right? Medicine has become modernized to meet our advancing lifestyles, right? If we were getting healthier and we were living life with a better quality than previously, the answers would be an astounding "Yes."

On one hand, we are living longer, no doubt. On the other hand, we, on average, are living with more disability, with more long-term-care facilities and with many more drug-dependent conditions which increase health care costs consistently. Medicare coverage is tightening more and more, as it is becoming prohibitively expensive to support the elderly population. Does insurance coverage offer us the assurance we need as we continue progressing? Progress is expensive. Money in insurance companies is dwindling, or so you would think based on the coverage offered to meet today's health needs.

As all technology progresses, we continue to enhance our lives through efficient means. Medical and surgical technologies parallel all other technological advancements. Medicine sustains lives today that otherwise would be lost, and is recognized among other heroic developments in our lifetime. As a result, we are indeed living longer. Life expectancy has reached an all-time high in the United States, with the average life expectancy being 77.6 years. As medicine continues to become modernized, we prolong life. At the same time, modern medicine has done nothing to increase the quality of life. This is where the problem lies. Quality of life enhancement does not fit into time-managed patient care.

In the insurance world, time is money. In the healing world, time is essential. They don't appear to go together. In addition, insurance companies continually need to change policies and have to protect their profit margins. So, while health care costs continually rise and insurance coverage becomes more restricted, the costs are passed along to the consumer in the form of higher premiums, co-pays and restricted medications. One simple example of this is a patient of mine who was required to have tubes put in his ears due to chronic ear infections. I treated his chronic ear infections with dietary changes, immune boosting supplements and ear drops. This particular patient hasn't had an ear infection since. Do you think that the insurance company paid for my services? Not in this case. Do you think my services saved the insurance company the cost of an outpatient surgery? Without question.

If we shift our focus to understanding the core health issues, and address them instead of placing a Band-Aid on them (which in essence causes a domino effect of more future problems), health care costs would ultimately drop. This is only one small part of the picture and not at all what this book is about. The bigger picture is a growing society that enjoys a greater quality of life, experiences more joy, has healthier relationships, makes better decisions, and experiences more peace and less chaos. Imagine how the planet at large would be affected if each of us individually, learn to and choose to be in this way. It's mind boggling to me, but my prayer nonetheless.

The world we live in is a reflection of what each of us carries around inside. Because so many people suffer physically or mentally or financially or romantically, this suffering billows out of our intimate worlds into every aspect of life that we touch. Our energy doesn't just live in our individual bodies. It expands beyond the physical body and impacts everyone we interact with on one level or another.

How do we attempt balance in the reality of our rapidly

advancing world? Think back to how simple life used to be. Remember how the discovery of electric light changed our lives forever? When traveling by airplane became possible, certain places became accessible that would otherwise remain out of the reach of most people. This one discovery changed many things in our interactive world. Now we have the World Wide Web, which connects us to the entire world instantly! These are but a few of the discoveries that, once they were established, we could never imagine doing without. Each time, an energy shift took place that affected all of us in a permanent way.

Medical practices are certainly not stagnant; rather, they continue to be modernized and improved, and become more efficient. I personally only carry medical insurance for catastrophic situations because this is where my faith in allopathic medicine lies. For chronic situations, I prefer to be under the care of someone who will listen to me, understand my challenges and work with me to assist the changes I need to make, to shift the direction my health is going in. Even in an acute, non-life-threatening condition, my preference is to work with someone who understands what my body needs to heal. The way I treat my body will acutely and ultimately influence the chronic condition of my being. If I'm in a car accident, or have an ectopic pregnancy requiring surgery, or have an airway obstruction, or require bypass surgery to save the life of my heart, I'll know that my insurance assures me that I will be covered financially.

If I suffered daily fatigue, headaches, PMS, irritable bowel syndrome, joint pain, depression, endometriosis, transitioning hormones, flu, cold, a minor sports injury, et cetera, my insurance coverage would not assure me that I was taken care of. As a Naturopathic Physician, I need to treat these conditions, when they occur in my patients, with more respect. A pill alone doesn't fix anything. A pill plus an understanding of the experience will not only prevent recurrence but it will maintain a forward motion in the manifestation of optimal health. All of this will make a great deal more sense as you continue reading.

Balancing our expansive nature with one that requires peace as a foundation becomes the focus of healing. Our intellect, creativity, desire, and passion are the foundations for anything conceivable. Our expanding world is addictive and absolutely amazing. Here is the question to ponder: "What price do we pay for the abandonment of simplicity?" The gains are obvious, but what about the losses?

Chapter 4

Medicine and Healing

How It Has Been Is Not How It Is

Historically there have been tribal healers and traditional medicine practices that addressed suffering in far different ways than we do today. Healing ceremonies reconnected people to both the earth and spiritual energy. Traditional practices routinely brought groups of people together, creating harmony and connectedness on many levels to facilitate healing. In our culture, we are devoid of these practices. There are many reasons for this. Because of the advent of the drug industry, we as a society know more about drugs than we do about herbs and homeopathy. The fast food chains have capitalized on people having little time, little money, and little education to understand the calorie-dense, nutrient-deficient nature of the food. We all carry cell phones around, making us available to the entire world at every moment. We can get a college degree by sitting in front of a computer rather than interacting with people and events on a one-on-one basis. It's odd, in a way. We have all these opportunities to be more connected, like through the Internet and with cell phones, but at the same time they act as barriers to shared human experience, rendering us all less connected to each other as well as to ourselves.

Recognize how, in the face of advancing technology, we experience the loss of the self on many levels. It is possible to put effort into reconnecting to the self in its perfection and simplicity even *more* deeply than before the connection was interrupted. How we reconnect to the self is what this book is all about. You will learn to tap into your unique resources—the very rich and exceedingly abundant opportunities within you that are yearning to unfold. The yearning parts of you are your symptoms. You will be invited to use your unique resources for all they're worth, to bite into this opportunity like an apple and love every bit of it.

If, as a world, we don't learn to come home to the self, making this a conscious choice—if we choose not to make ourselves available to our own healing and to each other's, chronic illness will become not just an epidemic but an expected lifestyle.

∞ Chapter 5 ∞

Medicine and Healing

∫

One Step at a Time

We were born with the five senses to interact with our world—touch, smell, sight, taste and hearing. These senses are receivers that translate the sensations of feeling good or bad. Think of all of the wonderful ways that you can nurture these God-given gifts to experience the emotion of joy. The most wonderful aspects of life are alive because of our senses. We experience colorful foods with varying textures served on delicately painted china with cloth napkins and crystal glasses holding water shining with the clarity of ice cubes. Not only does this presentation look pleasing, but it also makes the taste of the food more exquisite. We burn candles or keep fresh flowers to fill the air with enticing aromas. We will choose from our musical collection to fill the room with specific sounds to carry us more deeply into our intended experiences. None of us can deny the tenderness of the human touch. We've all had experiences as simple as scratching an itch. Imagine further the desire to receive a massage, to hold a baby, to feel the wind blowing through your hair, to hold hands, to achieve pure intimacy.

Along with the physical senses, we all have an intuitive sense like the gnawing in the stomach when you just know that something is wrong. You can get goose bumps when you just know something is right—like a thrill of excitement running through your body. You may have experienced times when you just sense something, but have no other physical or descriptive knowledge of this sense. You should not ignore this sense. Your five senses connect you to your physical world. Your intuitive sense connects you to wisdom within.

How many of our sense-fulfilling experiences are being compromised through our advancements? Instead of our advancements giving us more time to relax and enjoy our simple pleasures, they seem to be giving us more time to be busy! Because of this reality, we can now have sex over the Internet—gracious me! We can pull a frozen dinner out of the freezer on those days that we need the convenience. The convenience is mandatory to allow us to work later and get more done. We can continue working at our computers while the dinner is heating up in the microwave and then we can eat it without even tasting it as we type away! We miss precious time with the natural textures, colors and flavors of food preparation that involve cleaning and cutting and balancing flavors. But, as well, we miss out on the aromas and the flavors that cook together to create a symphony of taste that could never be captured in frozen food that is covered with plastic and nuked for a minute or so. Is there any wonder why our bodies are suffering?

This "lack of connectedness" that is given to us by fast foods, cell phones, and Internet technology, feeds a "lack of connectedness" to ourselves. The result is disconnection.

Healing then becomes very isolated. We are forced to become self-reliant. This requires a whole lot more energy, time, and money. It is, however, necessary to have come this far away from our true selves. The experience itself is providing for us the very opportunity to recognize our reality strongly enough to begin to do something about it.

Many, but certainly not all, people living today enjoy all of the advancements and growth of our world in all aspects. It's exhilarating to see the human potential that provided something different to experience today that wasn't available or even thought of yesterday. Each new experience lets us know that there are limitless other experiences that we haven't even tapped into yet. Our new experiences and opportunities are, however, inadvertently making us sick without our knowing it. This unknowingness is responsible for the chronic disease explosion.

We tend to react by default to the advancements of our world. We create disconnectedness simply by not keeping our awareness in our five senses or in our spiritual sense. By default, we do not realize whether or not we feel at ease or lack-of-ease. This default is unquestionably leading us to more illness. Illness is simply a manifestation in the physical body of lack-of-ease.

Our life progress does not have to create disharmony at all. We tend to think more about what we must do rather than focusing on who we are, in the moment of whatever it is we are doing. If, in this moment, you are conscious of nurturing and enriching the experience given you by your five senses and your spiritual sense, you are focusing on feeling great. If one sense organ is overstimulated, your focus tends to be more on what's stimulating it rather than on the part of you that feels good, and the balance is interrupted.

It is possible to bring enough foresight and action into our existence so that we do not have to pay for the gifts that our technology provides, by default, unconsciously. We all have the potential to react to our ever-expansive, ever-changing reality with balance, consciously. The goal is to resist the natural tendency to become disconnected and instead choose to create experiences that are even more fulfilling. As rhythms of our daily living shift, we can create harmony in the new rhythms that can be even more satisfying. It's not just that we can, we must. We must create the harmony, as it doesn't happen effortlessly. We create the harmony by first becoming conscious of where each of us has personally evolved to right now. Ask yourself if you are at ease, enjoying all of your life? Are you enjoying your relationships, from intimate ones to parent-child ones to colleagues to friends? Do you enjoy your line of work? Do you enjoy your physical body, its health and vitality? Do you enjoy your time off? Do you enjoy your alone time?

Bring your consciousness to your reality and look at what might need a little more attention. Are you living life in the fast lane and loving it? Do you wish you could slow down and have more time off? Do you wish you had more things to do with your time? Each of us will answer these questions personally, and if you feel good answering the questions, you are on the right track. If you don't feel good as you answer these questions, you need to give conscious awareness to shifting whatever is necessary so that you do feel good about answering them. Use all of your senses, from the tangible to the intangible to reflect on these questions. Let your mind relax and let the sensations within you do the answering. Feel your answer rather than think your answer. This is the way to utilize your greatest sense.

Being unaware of the changes that you may need to make in order to adjust to the ever-changing world allows you only one option: that is, to live by default. So many people have not "advanced with the advancements," and end up paying the price of compromised health. "Advancing with the advancements," to me, means that you get all of the benefits of the wonderful technology that has sped our lives up without compromising your inner peace. This is a feasible endeavor.

I believe the phenomenon of chronic disease, which is the result of our disconnection, to be the journey that brings us back together as individuals and as a society.

The very first step in healing is recognition. The second step is choosing healthy experiences based on your recognition. The third step is to get direct feedback from the body as to whether you are on track or not and to make the necessary changes to be on track. This book will help you learn how to follow these simple steps to healing, creating ease in your life.

Healing = Ease

Recognize if you are at ease or not.

Choose experiences that allow you to feel at ease.

∞ Chapter 6 ∞

Medicine and Healing

∫

The One on One Experience

In my practice as a naturopathic physician, I find it of the utmost importance to always meet a person where they are in their healing journey. If someone desires a medication to treat their symptoms, I will honor this. If someone needs a surgical referral, I will recommend this. I don't cast spells, wear beaded clothing, or mix brews that your family is to share at midnight facing north to summon your guides for healing. Although rituals sound fun, this is not where my patients are at.

I refer to chronic illness repeatedly throughout this book, and it is true that I frequently meet a patient for the first time who lets me know that I am his or her last hope.

He or she has been everywhere, been worked up head to toe and nothing identifiable or treatable has yet been revealed. The other half of the time, my clinical practice brings to me very high-functioning people who are looking for a quick fix. And of course this is the case, as it reflects the world we live in. While addressing patients' needs, even the quick-fix-seekers, I like to take time to educate each person about the symbol of their illness. Each person's symptoms are simply what opened the door to an understanding of his or her underlying condition.

Regardless of the individual's healing experience, I find the entire healing process fascinating, as time after time, it is the same. We all need to reconnect to ourselves and to our world. We bounce around like ping pong balls, flitting here, flitting there. Bounce, bounce, bounce.

What if we had a traditional practice that we came home to, to share with our family and close friends? What if we made time to nurture each other and share in rituals? So many families don't even sit down together to eat dinner at the end of the day. Parents, often both, are working later, kids are filling their lives with more and more activities, but if they are home, they're on the Game Cube—nurturing that expanding, thinking mind! Think of the games that kids play. They have a controller in their laps with buttons and knobs to move objects on the television screen. They may be running, fighting, or driving cars in a race. The excitement and energy are being manipulated through these knobs. The body is still, the excitement is high, and there is no outlet for their bodies. Aggressive energy gets locked up in their little bodies and minds. Then what?

If we had enough peaceful downtime at home, we

wouldn't need a chronic illness to make us a candidate for disability. We wouldn't need chronic pain so that we could take painkillers to numb us to our worlds. We wouldn't need diet drinks to replace overindulged calories from unbalanced eating. We wouldn't need so many sleeping pills to knock us out of our ever-thinking, ever-fixing, ever-worrying and chattering monkey-mind at night. We wouldn't need meds to give us a functioning sex life!

Perhaps you may share in a weekly religious ceremony of going to church or temple. This is a ritual. I find each and every religion fascinating. It is an excellent opportunity to connect with others and to support each other in a belief system. It is very honoring and loving to everyone in the group. What happens if you're not in the group? You'll probably go to hell. What? Come on, people! Oh, tradition based in fear. Sign me up.

I don't think this epidemic of chronic disease is due to lack of enough antidepressants or lack of knowledge. I believe it to be a symbol of our lack of connection to ourselves and others. True healing requires love. Love of self. Love of your life. Love of your relationships. Love of the choices you've made. Love of the opportunities you have. Would you be sick if love were the foundation of your entire life? The problem exists because we're not taught how to create this for ourselves.

∞ Chapter 7 ∞

Medicine and Healing

∫

The Naturopathic Medical Approach

The field of naturopathic medicine's approach is to teach people how to create healing. The first step taught in naturopathic medicine is "remove the cause." Is your relationship bringing you harm? Is your job bringing you harm? Is your diet bringing you harm?

This first step of healing is very nice, isn't it? Regardless of how nice it is, not many of my patients are willing up front to address this first step. I find that eventually, if individuals stay connected to the process of healing, they look the bull in the eyes. This process often takes time, occasionally it's quick, and other times it never happens. This is why

I believe that healing is a very personal event, as it is guided by the individual—on their time, when they're ready.

The patients that I commonly treat come in with a specific agenda. If I'm not helping them meet their agenda, I'm out of the conversation and they're onto the next physician who can or can't help them. If a person comes into my office obviously suffering from allergies, it will be difficult for him to embrace a diet of vegetables and fish if he is used to eating emotionally when he does not feel well. It would be healing to have him take time off to relax and drink teas while a hot castor oil pack lies over his liver. Since he only knows life in the fast lane, this approach probably won't translate very well. He may hear the importance of changing his diet to decrease systemic inflammation, and to slow down to heal, but he may not be able to endure the time and restrictions without some acute therapy to assist him to feel better.

My medical privileges as a physician allow me to get on the journey with people, but it is my philosophy that directs the journey. My philosophy is that healing is uniquely individual and, when combined with joy, is a limitless experience.

∞ Chapter 8 ∞

Medicine and Healing

∫

Difficult but Simple

Conventional medicine focuses on keeping the body alive. By nature it is fear-based. Naturopathic medicine focuses on the quality of life while alive. By nature it is love-based. I do believe that through love, honor and respect of the self we absolutely can live longer lives, but this isn't the focus. The focus is on quality. None of us know when our last day will be, but we all know whether or not we are happy.

Many books have defined love and fear as the only two categories of emotion, under which all other emotions fall. Any definitive emotion that opposes love is categorized as fear, while any emotion that opposes fear is categorized as love. Since illness and wellness are opposite experiences, illness would be defined as a fearful experience and wellness would be defined as a love-based experience. If you simply think of being ill, the emotion of fear has the potential to surface and if you think of being well, the emotion of love has the potential to surface. Since conventional medicine focuses on treating illnesses it is, by definition, fear-based. It is focused on fixing problems. Naturopathic medicine focuses on *refocusing* as a foundation to healing. For example, if you focus on your fatigue as a problem, it is stuck. If you can refocus your fatigue from an unwanted symptom to a specific way your body is getting your attention to slow down and take time to explore how you are spending your energy, it is not a problem; rather, it is a gift. If you consider your symptoms as merely problems, it is impossible to attach the emotion of love to them.

Naturopathic Medical Doctors recognize that the symptom being treated didn't just occur today. The human body is very good at compensating and adjusting biochemical and physiological pathways and experiences to create homeostasis. Homeostasis means a stable, steady state (*homeo* = similar, *stasis* = stable state) and is exactly what the body does day after day in all experiences. Over time, the body becomes less and less efficient at creating homeostasis, as it takes more energy and resources that are no longer available to keep the body in balance.

Once the body can no longer adjust to maintain harmony, symptoms begin to surface. These symptoms are given names, or diagnoses. This is where allopathic medicine intervenes—at the level of the diagnosis. It treats the endpoint. This is why it is fear-based.

If the endpoint is not life threatening, it is more of a

nuisance than anything. Your doctor may have the answer to remove this nuisance. To do so, it may take a medication to manipulate your system to either not notice the nuisance or surgery to actually remove the nuisance. We are fooling ourselves if we think we are well at this point, but most people do. The path that got you to this endpoint is the focus of Naturopathic Medicine. This is why it is love-based.

I have noticed that as we mature as a culture, more and more people are becoming aware that they really do want more than just a Band-Aid or a suppressive treatment in non-emergency situations. I certainly do prescribe antidepressants for chronic conditions, but *most often* I don't stop there. I stress *most often* because not every patient is ready for anything else at that time. However, I know that I'm in their healing path, and that the right experience will present itself at the right time.

Drug companies are aware of the American public wanting more from their doctors, which is one of the reasons that drug companies are now paying top dollar for television advertising. Medical care is becoming very patient-driven. While the American public is demanding more out of the medical profession to enhance the quality of their lives, there is a lot more dissatisfaction as their exact needs are not being met. We may have less burning in our stomachs because we are turning off the acid with the little purple pill, but we are also not absorbing our nutrients from food and therefore feeling even more tired. And who cares about the increased risk of heart attacks as long as we're able to enjoy a good sex life!

Our life challenges not only mirror our health challenges, but they also contribute to them. We advance in technology to stay more connected to our world, yet there is a definite level of disconnectedness. We enjoy medical advancements to immediately take our symptoms away, without taking the time to address the cause of the imbalance. Problem = Band-Aid. Then one day, we try to cover up the problem and it doesn't work. Or, we cover up the problem but cannot tolerate the side effects. All of a sudden, we don't have a clue why we are feeling a certain way!

It is not easy to look at your whole life and, in a brief moment, understand the influence it has had on your health. Healing requires slowing down now and opening to your knowingness inside. It requires breaking patterns of destruction, which of course must be understood before you can change them. It requires exploring what you love more than what is needed to survive. You may be a person who must first learn what you don't love before you learn what you do love, but knowing what you love and what you want are essential. If we all begin to relax and choose to enjoy all things, our hearts will open to knowing what we need individually to begin healing and to prevent familial tendencies towards disease.

The healing process is by no means easy. I encourage you to not get stuck needing things to be easy. In fact, don't even use the word in your vocabulary because it doesn't matter if it's easy or difficult. The road to success is keeping it simple. And so it is.

Inventory Time

Stop for a moment. Regardless of your current age, how do you feel with each passing day? How do you feel about your health? How do you feel about the world you have created for yourself? Do you lie awake at night wondering how you will lose those few extra pounds or what magic panacea will give you the level of energy that you want to feel? Do you compare yourself to others and wonder how they seem to have it all while you seem to struggle with getting a job or finding a passionate relationship—or any relationship, for that matter? You may be one of the lucky ones who is simply grateful for the absolute perfection of your life. You may already create naturally balanced health by making effortless choices that facilitate optimal wellness, passionate love and complete abundance without the feeling that you are sacrificing anything, from food to time to relationships. If your health is optimal but doesn't feel effortless, what part of you is being sacrificed? The answer to this question depends on what you define as a sacrifice. Is the chocolate more of a sacrifice than the depressed or manic energy you may feel in two hours? Is it easier for you to swallow your opinion in order to maintain a relationship in its current form or to speak your feelings and risk it changing, possibly dissolving or growing deeper?

∞ Chapter 9 ∞

Medicine and Healing

∫

A Chronic Problem

An article in the Journal of the American Medical Association dated September 1, 2004 states, "Chronic disease is now the principal cause of disability and use of health care services and consumes 78% of health expenditures." The article goes on to say, "We have [neither] trained our doctors to deal with this problem nor to provide those adequate therapeutic tools to meet the need."

It has been argued by allopathic physicians in the United States that the research on natural products typically performed overseas does not meet the "rigorous standards" of the United States. This is a clear example of how, if naturopathic physicians compete to become equals to allopathic physicians, we have to play by the same rules and follow the same standards to be accepted. I do not find it at all necessary to compete. Naturopathic medicine is unique in its approach, in its philosophy, and in its focus, just as allopathic medicine is unique in its approach, philosophy and focus. The language of healing must change for it to make any sense. Naturopathic Physicians recognize that cancer is a chronic condition—one that doesn't go away just because the space-occupying lesion that defines it is no longer in the body for a certain number of years. I find the word "cure" to be very misleading in either body of medicine.

It is impossible to attempt to design appropriate research projects meeting the standards that are acceptable to physicians in the United States to show any significance of true healing modalities, because healing is so multifaceted and so personal. A healthy body is one where all organ systems are in harmony with each other. Not only does our overall health reflect the complexities of our lifestyles, but also, individual organ health affects each of the other organs in our system.

It is possible, however, to design research projects to identify the benefits and risks of certain modalities such as botanical medicine if other aspects of the human experience are not manipulated or controlled. This type of research that provides information about the tools being used in the healing process is both interesting and very important, yes. Unfortunately most of these necessary studies are not done because the financial investment is less than the financial gain in providing evidence of the benefits of an unpatentable substance.

On this note, did you know that the research that is done on medication is done by the very drug company that is formulating and selling the drug? The results are presented to the Food and Drug Administration (FDA), which decides whether the drug is approved for its intended use or not.

It's an unfortunate truth that the opponents of naturopathic medicine define our specialty as weak due to lack of research, when unmet chronic illnesses consume 78% of health care dollars. The statistics today would be very different if the money spent to keep illnesses in the system were spent on healing modalities that make common sense, even though they don't have double-blind, placebo controlled, randomized testing to back them up.

Furthermore, due to the complex human experience, medicine has labeled "undiagnosable" chronic diseases as syndromes or as conditions with a psychological origin. Syndromes are conditions that are diagnosed by exclusion, meaning there is no concrete evidence to point to a specific disease pathology but there are a certain number of symptoms occurring simultaneously in an individual. Since there is no diagnosable pathology, it must be coming from the person's head. Ah-hah! Our mind may play a very important role in healing.

Without question, the health-disease continuum is multifaceted. The conversation at large becomes centered on how to reestablish a sense of balance. There are many, many potential paths to achieving balance. Hence, I do not think any one medical practice or therapy is the answer. We are complex beings. Our options are many. As I stated earlier, we need to allow all things and our hearts will open to our personal healing process.

In summary, the conventional medical model isn't evolving quickly enough to sustain the demands of today's people. It is providing quick fixes, but there is a price to pay for this. Conventional medical doctors are great at what they do—honor them for that! Now, to answer the questions you may have about chronic fatigue, depression, anxiety, cancer, insomnia and pain, as well as your desire to optimize your quality of life through efforts such as anti-aging, hormonal balancing, and sports enhancement, you need to seek professionals trained in dealing with these issues. The frustration exists because the *right questions are being asked of the wrong person.*

∞ Chapter 10 ∞

Medicine and Healing

∫

Evolution

It is important to expand upon our understanding of how our health care has not sufficiently addressed chronic ailments, while at the same time extending our life expectancies. Why wouldn't we be seeking opportunities to slow down the aging process to enjoy these extra years? As we evolve, we need the medical model to evolve with us. Naturopathic medicine provides this. Naturopathic medicine offers opportunities to people to approach health from a new perspective. The naturopathic colleges are actively graduating physicians and the state licensing boards issue hundreds of licenses to Naturopathic Medical Doctors

(NMDs) each year. The profession itself is getting much larger and it is my hope that it will become stronger as well.

All things in medicine change slowly—the approval of new drugs, new diagnostic testing or new surgical procedures takes years to manifest. Students and physicians of naturopathic medicine today are striving to be recognized and respected in the medical arena, and therefore look to the standards of conventional medicine as guidelines. If the goal is for naturopathic physicians to be accepted on an equal basis with conventional physicians as primary care doctors, it would be necessary for us to be similar to the conventional doctors so that a comparison could be made, right? To accept equally you need to compare like to like. So, politically and respectfully, the profession at large is on a quest for standardization of naturopathy. It is my hope that we won't get all excited and start fighting for the wrong things!

This very thing happened to doctors of osteopathy (DOs) when they wanted to be recognized as a body of medicine equal to medical doctors (MDs) and lost their philosophy of the spine as the center of health in the body. The foundational philosophy of DO schools was centered on spinal health. Most DOs today don't even think of the spine! I certainly am not judging DOs as less legitimate physicians—I just find it sad that they have lost their roots in their founding philosophy. Unfortunately, for the profession to survive, DOs needed to exercise the same privileges with their patients as MDs did. Training in pharmacology and surgery offered them the same privileges. So, why has their philosophy become lost? It takes time to educate people. It takes time for patients to adopt a new living philosophy. Insurance companies aren't ready to pay for this time, yet. Bravo for insurance companies though, for paying for spinal manipulation by chiropractic physicians, DO's, and NMDs for the treatment of personal injury claims! This is a great first step in the recognition of non-surgical care for structural injuries. The next step is to have them pay for spinal manipulation for the prevention of degenerative processes. This is a good sign that we're on the right track.

So when insurance companies come to my door to sign me up as a provider on their plans, along come guidelines that I must follow. Ten minutes is allowed for this condition, five for that. If you "label" or diagnose this condition, only these labs will be covered. Baloney! Of course there need to be rules to follow so everyone is on the same page, but these rules do not fit in individualized medicine. It takes a lot of time to play by all of the rules, time I'd rather be spending with my patients.

Once I sacrifice my philosophy, I forfeit my potential to truly make a difference. If I wanted to be a conventional physician, I would have done that. I'd rather go to one when I need one.

I believe that we begin to get sick as we separate ourselves from what we love. My passion lies in observing the human potential. Naturopathic medicine offers me the opportunity to influence the human potential to heal. Do I have a 100% track record? Absolutely not! No physician does.

Naturopathic medical doctors are recognized as family practitioners with a specialty in naturopathic medicine. Insurance companies lack the guidelines to offer coverage for our care. In the future, I believe it will be imperative for insurance companies to have a plan for NMDs. Health care is patient-driven and patients are demanding it. The statistics indicate a need to address the chronic ailments. We have come a long way, and I know there is progress with insurance companies already. My main hope is that as we continue advancing as a profession, we do not sacrifice our philosophy. There is no need to compete with conventional doctors. What we offer is different. Patients don't have to decide between an allopathic physician and a naturopathic physician. We need to respect when time calls for each one.

You know by now that naturopathic medicine is much more than employing an herb rather than a drug. It does include a journey of healing with minimal use of medications and surgery to manipulate the body's systems, but it is much broader than this, and much more interesting.

Healing is different from suppression or removal. Suppressing symptoms and removing tumors, lesions and even organs focuses on the pathology—the end result. This is what conventional medicine does well. Naturopathic medicine treats the physiology. We treat what is happening right now that is allowing the pathology to manifest. The patient intake is much different—lifestyle, nutrition practices, elimination patterns, exercise, stress level and one's management of it all—all of this is important, as each of these choices affects our biochemistry and physiology, manifesting either in pathology or optimal health.

Our interest is in what journey takes us to this last outcome. The journey manifests in all three bodies—the "physical body," the emotional or "mind-body," and the "spiritual body." In true healing, all three bodies must be addressed at some point. Naturopathic medicine honors the whole person. Symptoms are merely symbols of how our imbalance is being expressed.

∞ Chapter 11 ∞

Medicine and Healing

∫

Where Do You Fit?

This book is designed to help you see how you fit—in your body, in your world, and in your healing process. The mind-body-spirit approach offers three distinctive areas to put your energy into. You will notice that in giving attention to one aspect of the self, all aspects are influenced. Healing is a beautiful, honorable journey that takes awareness and action. At the same time, optimal wellness is a very personal definition. Your level of optimal wellness is defined by you.

So, you have the idea. We are evolving and changing as individuals and as a society. How can we be the best we can be because of our advancements, not in spite of them?

We have so many tools to guide our journey of healing. We have acupuncture, chelation, drugs, herbs, homeopathy, nutritional support, physical medicine (manipulation, massage, and hydrotherapy), reflexology, subconscious reprogramming, surgery, and so on. I put them in alphabetical order because no one is more important than the others. Tools are vehicles. Whichever one resonates within the relationship between the patient and physician is the right one for that experience.

Okay. We have the patient, we have the doctor, we have the symptom or condition, we have the tools—now what? Now the journey begins.

∞ Chapter 12 ∞

The Mind

∫

Healing the Mind-Body Relationship

Notice that you are always in relationship to your body. You might love it and speak silent, beautiful words to it every day. You might hate it and speak ugly, demanding things to it every day. Your relationship to your body may not be a conscious awareness. Stop for a moment, and bring your awareness into your body. Notice how you feel about your physical body. You may have a strong emotion towards it or you may be so disconnected from it that you don't feel a thing. The important thing to know is that it really doesn't matter what you notice. Give yourself permission to simply notice without any judgment.

What you notice is not good or bad, right or wrong. What does matter is your awareness. Without awareness nothing can happen. At the same time, awareness with judgment is absolutely and totally worthless.

If that paragraph felt like going on a rollercoaster—hold on! Healing is just that—unwinding the very patterns that keep us stuck. The most obstructive form of thought is judgment. Anyone reading this book is looking for guidance to heal on some level. Whatever your concern or condition is, recognize how you judge yourself for it. "I'm too fat, I'm too tired, I'm too sick, I'm too old." Notice your tone as well and how your body feels when you play these judgments over and over and over in your monkey mind.

Healing the physical body requires the highest level of respect. If you have any judgment of yourself, there is a level of respect missing. "But," you'll say, "I like 'such and such' about myself." There are simple rules to live by as you step into your healing journey. First—no "buts," no "I don't knows," no "shoulds," no "never or always"— these words should disappear from your vocabulary forever! It's okay if you forget and sneak these words into your everyday language—as long as you catch yourself and start over. Respect feels a whole lot better than coercion. Compare "I should stop eating wheat" to "I give myself permission to choose what my body needs to stay healthy." As respect enters the equation of health, things get easier, they mean more, and the results stick.

It's amazing how your body responds to your internal dialogue. We're speaking of the physical body here, so let's bring in a little physics. Physics is the law of understanding how the physical world relates to the energetic world. The connection is constant and always moving. The constant movement offers endless possibilities. You directly affect this energy through everything that you think, say and do. You decide how you will interact with your world. Your world does not manipulate you. Actually, I take that back: your world does manipulate you, if you allow it to. This is what victimization and complacency are. If you are connected to your center, your source, and your power, your world will not manipulate you; it will reflect you.

Your physical body, which is the part that is most likely guiding you to heal, is the world in which your spirit, soul, emotions and thoughts live. Your body is the house for the intangible you. It is the physical package of the non-physical. Your body is your physical world. So, every conversation you have affects your body. Physics is the science of matter and energy and of the interactions between the two. Hence, we all have a physical manifestation of the balance of all of our bodies—physical, emotional-mental, spiritual.

So, now you are realizing that your body is merely the physical space. This space is *animated* by your non-physical space. Isn't that a marvelously illuminating perspective of the physical body? This gives you permission to lighten up on your physical body—to change any negative belief that you have about your body. Instead of telling your body that it is so tired or in so much pain or is so weak, tell it instead that it is doing a great job giving you feedback! The feedback you are getting is about your non-physical body. Your thoughts animate your body. Our thoughts create our emotions. Our emotions create our feelings. Our feelings are felt or perceived in the physical body.

The mind-emotional body is an intertwined body that makes choices (thoughts) based on its feelings (emotions). They cannot be separated. It is impossible to make a choice without an emotion attached to it. Even stoic people who express few to no emotions are linked to their non-emotion while making decisions. The choices you make and the motivations behind your choices are big components of the roadmap of your body. Are your choices opening doors or closing doors? Are you choosing to live in honor of life or in destruction of it? Each and every choice affects our physiology—not just the food that we eat, not just the drugs that we take, not just the genes we inherit—everything impacts the physiology, the physical body, including the choices that we make in our lives.

When I started writing this book, I began with the physical body. Everything I was writing first had to do with the power of choice. Choosing good food, choosing healthy relationships, et cetera . . . I do value educating people about optimal nutrition and herbs and such matters, but I find that emotions dictate choices much more so than intellect does. In clinical practice it's important to know what people are eating and how they are exercising. I'm much more interested, however, in why they are choosing certain things over others. Our decisions are *very* emotionally based. The first step in healing, then, is not learning about their condition; rather, it is recognizing self-respect. Respect influences self-care and compliance with a healing program more than does the information one learns in the program. Therefore, the very choices you make about how to treat your physical body are emotionally driven and tend to be more the issue in healing than the knowledge of what is optimal for your body.

Notice Your Story

Think of a time recently when you made a decision for yourself that was not respectful. Perhaps it was a time that you chose to mindlessly eat a food that wasn't good for you. Maybe you were in conversation with a loved one and you didn't say what you wanted to. Or, maybe you impulsively went on a shopping spree and ended up with things you didn't need. You choose the experience; any one will do.

Now, write down the whole experience, starting from what was going on right before it. Perhaps you were bored, or you just had a disagreement with someone. Or maybe you were silently having a dialogue with yourself about how you were lazy or fat or boring or stressed. Write it all down as though you were writing a story about it for someone else to read. Finish your story with how you felt after the experience.

Go back and read it over and underline each and every sentence that you wrote that reflected a lack of self-respect.

Rewrite your story, this time changing the underlined sentences to ones that reflect self-respect. As you write the new story, have FUN! See yourself actually making these choices. Notice how the story and life experience could have been very different than they were.

Use this information to make different choices tomorrow.

Example of Noticing My Story

I leave my office by 1:45 each day to pick up my son from school. Inevitably <u>something happens at work to delay my</u> leaving and therefore <u>I stress</u> to get to him on time. Once we are in the house, I get him a snack. This day, I started <u>eating Goldfish by the fistfuls</u>. I <u>didn't even taste</u> them. <u>I didn't even notice I was doing this until I was stuffed</u>! My stomach felt so heavy and uncomfortable. I looked at the bag and noticed how much I had eaten and <u>felt gross</u>. <u>Afterwards I felt cranky and lacked the desire to play and have fun with my kids and wasn't even able to share in my interaction with them. Each time I notice my full stomach, I remember what a loser I was</u> for eating all those Goldfish.

I leave my office by 1:45 each day to pick up my son from school. I will not allow anything to get in my way of getting him on time. Once we are in the house, I get him a snack. As I am preparing this for him, I prepare in my mind a snack that is more appropriate for me and physically prepare it when I am done with his. I sit down with him and taste every bite. I eat only enough to make me feel good. Afterwards I feel energetic and joyful when playing with my kids. I am present to the entire experience. Each time I notice my body, I remember how well I take care of it.

∞ Chapter 13 ∞

The Mind

∫

Learning to Love

Over the past nine years of practice I have become fascinated by observing the power that our mind has over our bodies. There are a limitless number of belief systems and motivations that govern our day-to-day choices. What is mind-boggling to me is the effect that each of these choices has on our biochemistry.

There is such a subtle exchange of information that is constantly going on between our minds and our bodies. I will use a personal example to demonstrate this delicate, ever-adjusting balance. One day it was time for me to put my oldest son to bed. Just prior to our bedtime snack I became upset with something he had done. (The real kicker here is that I can't for the life of me remember what it was that he did, and this happened only about a month ago. So, not only is the message in this story so poignant, it reminds me of how trivial the events that shape our lives truly are!) Okay, so here I was now sitting at the kitchen table, alone, not speaking, with my arms angrily folded across my chest. Since it had been so quiet for so long, I decided to use a tool that I teach people to use each day to manifest what they desire in their lives.

Silently I asked for help with this situation. I asked myself, "If love were my only option right now and I chose it, what would happen here?" Clear as day, I heard: "Just love him." And as clear as day I heard myself answer, "Nope." I was too angry to follow through. So, he proceeded to bed and so did I. We skipped the reading and back patting that is typical for our bedtime ritual. I couldn't sleep a wink that night. I felt dreadfully immature and irresponsible as a parent. I take parenting responsibilities seriously in order to teach our children to be the best they can be. In my opinion we are the best we can be only when we are functioning from a perspective of love—and I couldn't choose love with my innocent seven-year-old child! I snuck into his room while he was sleeping to kiss him and rub his back, and I couldn't wait for him to wake up so that I could apologize to him.

The lesson here is that at the moment that I lacked the courage to follow through and open to love, my biochemistry changed—I couldn't sleep, I felt tight and inflexible and the next day was a waste because of the lack of sleep I had the night before. It became very clear to me, at that very moment, just how deeply our cells are affected by our choices. Bam! Right there, I went into lockdown mode emotionally and physically. There is such a definite and strong connection there. I hope that through this story you can begin to recognize this truth that exists between your mind and your body and just how deeply your cells respond to your life choices. Imagine, once we all begin to respect this and all of our choices are born from love, how the energy of our world will begin to shift.

The only reason that we feel the need to fight is because we are insecure and this is our form of self-protection. What if your cells didn't have the need to feel protected? How would your conversations and relationships be different? What if you chose to believe that all is as it should be and all is well? This comes from Louise Hay's teaching. All is as it should be and all is well. Does this not open your body up to freedom, ease, grace and peace? Feel your body move into the belief that all is as it should be and all is well. There is no fight. When there is no fight, we get out of our own way.

This whole notion of insecurity and fighting specifically feeds our belief that competition is a necessary part of life. Competition can certainly be healthy as it assists us in becoming the best that we can become. Competition can also be unhealthy, as it brings a tremendous amount of discord between us and others and, quite frankly, it brings discord within our own selves! How often have you committed to eating healthier, only to fail at your commitment within three days? You are competing with your will and your will lost. Your dialogue over time will change to, "Oh, what's the use?" You've given in to something else that won, not you. You don't particularly like this thing that won and you feel powerless before it.

I'd like us to take the time to really observe competition

in our lives and how it is the biggest opponent of love. If we are in competition for one thing, there will always be disappointment on one side. If, on the other hand, as we are competing, we realize that there are many ways to win, both sides win. We can win by having an attitude that we are here to have fun, to learn, and to continue improving. The trophy is the endpoint. In life there is never an endpoint, but we live as though there were, especially when we are competing. What a waste of time. Our personal competitive nature is determined by our perspective of life. For example, death can be viewed as an endpoint and/or a beginning point. It depends on your point of view of life. I remember hearing Dr. Christiane Northrup at one of her workshops saying, "Birth and death are really the same thing; the only difference is who is waiting for you on the other side." Again, we create our life based on our own perspective. Why not choose a perspective that feels good?

Let's focus back on the unhealthy aspect which I define as competing for one thing and one thing only—one trophy, one award, one sum of money, one outcome. Remember that out of competition arises insecurity and fighting. Nothing could be more opposite to the practice of love than insecurity within our own hearts and fighting with the people who have ordinarily been good friends or family members. Unhealthy competition *anywhere* in our life is one of our biggest challenges to living peacefully and joyfully.

Understanding the finesse of competition will bring clarity to your practice in self-love and will be reflected in the love of your entire world. Contemplate an experience where two people are opposing one another, perhaps in a tennis match. You are the spectator and have a bond with one of the players. You have totally aligned with him and support him, respect him, and honor him. Whatever the outcome of the game is, you will have a particular emotion connected with it. If, on the other hand you were more aligned with the other player, your emotional reaction would be entirely different. So if you stand back and look at the two people opposing one another, recognize that you can choose to align your energy with either one—equally. This leaves room for understanding that both are really very good. Both players deserve equal respect from all people, not just those who are "on their side," so to speak.

The reality of the times that we live in now is that our belief in competition is losing its finesse and becoming more of an instinctual response, because we are defining one outcome as our only focus. In our primitive world, competition was a necessary instinct for the purpose of survival. The human race, however, has evolved in its level of intellectual and emotional complexity. As we have evolved into our current state of being we have become sophisticated in many ways. Primitive guttural sounds have evolved into words of many languages. Movements and postures have become graceful and elegant. Emotional bonds possess intimacy and pride rather than survival value. As we have become emotionally intellectual beings, we have somehow also carried forward the primitive belief in competition for survival. This lack of refinement, in my opinion, is responsible for the degeneration of the sophistication that we have adapted to.

Competition as an instinct rather than a respected exchange for the betterment of all is an unevolved form.

Healing 101 65

The result is *unhealthy* competition which interferes with self-love. As we "evolve," competition is becoming more and more unhealthy because fear is embedding itself in many consciousnesses. Let's create a picture of healthy competition. Consider a respectful sporting event as a display of the masterful beauty of physical strength and control, with good sportsmanship and the knowledge that all players applied their very best regardless of the outcome. Each player is grateful for the other, for without him or her there would be no game. Each player demonstrates their masterful physical skill and perfected physique because of the other player or players. There is an element of respect that is necessary to maintain the enjoyment of the game from the perspective of the players as well as from that of the spectators.

Competition in our daily world certainly lacks this poise. Imagine if each one of us chose to only compete in this manner. Growing and becoming better at what we do *because* of each other, rather than *in spite* of each other? Why do you think that we don't do this naturally? I think the answer is simple . . . we are not taught this. Nowadays disrespectful competition begins at a very early age. I felt it clearly at my five-year-old's soccer game! Angry parents were making angry kids because the kids didn't get the ball or run fast enough or win the game. I was pleased however that it wasn't our team displaying the lack of sportsmanship—so we must have attracted players on our team as a reflection of the group consciousness and attracted the competitive team to remind us of what we don't want to be. It was so clear. Regardless, I don't remember this amount of parental bull when I was a kid. Are we evolving faster and faster towards our own destruction? Indeed. Does it have to be this way? Indeed not.

It may seem small and insignificant, but what if, one at a time, we all chose to interact in a loving manner—towards each other and towards the event itself? Remember how much we influence each other from our internal energy point? A domino effect begins to happen. I don't see that we have any other option. Destruction or liberation—it is determined by all of us.

In order for us to practice the exercise in living in love at all times, we start by understanding these concepts and how energy exchanges that occur within us are ultimately reflected in our complete world. Begin noticing what makes you feel good and what makes you feel bad. When you feel bad inside, practice opening up to what feels good. You will only be able to practice this once you become more clear on what it is you are feeling at all times.

Feel Your Story

Think of a recent experience that was difficult for you.

Close your eyes and play the whole thing in your mind as if you were watching a video of the whole scenario. Watch the details closely. Remember where you were, who you were with, what the conversation was, et cetera. Watch this movie of you in your life as if it were happening again right now.

As you are watching the most challenging part of that experience, notice how your body feels. Notice clearly what your body is experiencing.

Whatever you notice—tight stomach, holding breath, aching head, tight fists—this is *where* your emotion is living in your body.

Lastly, be grateful to your body.

Notice the body part that got your attention. Thank it directly for getting your attention so clearly and so immediately. You can do this silently or out loud. The only thing that matters is that you end this exercise with gratitude—gratitude that your body got your attention.

∞ Chapter 14 ∞

The Mind

$$\int$$

Choosing Love

Your complete awareness of self allows you to recognize how much self-respect you have. When you recognize that you are not feeling good by noticing resistance in your body, notice that this is just a signal to you that in that particular moment, you are choosing something that is disrespectful of your being. That's all. And by noticing, you have the ability to make a different choice. My hope is that the exercise of the previous chapter becomes a daily practice for you. Recognition and awareness are always the first steps to creating something new or different. Consciously begin noticing experiences in your life that are not respectful to yourself. Once you start noticing these times, you can begin examining them more closely—if not at the time, then perhaps that night.

For example, if you are being spoken to disrespectfully, you have a few choices. One, you can match the person's energy and speak with anger back to the person to protect yourself. (This only fuels the fire of anger and is a no-win.) Two, you can swallow the comments and ignore them, changing the subject quickly. (This is a form of suppression of anger which if done repeatedly turns into depression.) Three, you can pause with the conversation, notice how you feel when you hear the words that the other person speaks, and speak from that feeling rather than from your head or ego that desperately wants to protect you. (This is an example of self-respect, self-love.) In this case, the conversation might sound like: "Excuse me for just a moment. I don't feel good when you speak to me in that manner."

This is the first step in healing—recognition and awareness. Recognition of experiences and patterns that you are choosing that lack self-respect. Once you've recognized patterns that are not in harmony with your being, you can begin to shift them into patterns that are in harmony with you.

The exercise in the previous chapter helped you to see just where you hold your challenging emotions and what they feel like. Begin to realize that your symptoms are knocks on the door. It's your body wanting you to pay attention. You're beginning to pay attention to your life experiences as well as to their effect on your body. Your physical reaction or symptom is energy in your body that is not at ease. Your body is experiencing lack of ease or dis-ease. Energy in your body that is not smooth and peaceful challenges your optimal cellular functioning. Your biochemistry and physiology are changing to patterns that oppose homeostasis. Homeostasis, as I discussed before, is a medical term that means everything is balanced and at ease.

I hope you are beginning to see that what you are doing as you practice these exercises is treating the *cause* of your symptoms. Medications that suppress your symptoms suppress your life if that is the end of your treatment plan. Medications—used properly—can enhance the quality of your life if your condition itself is so compromising that you have no quality at all. So, there is a place for medications to assist the journey of self-love as it often offers a person with a debilitating situation an opportunity to get a glimpse of how life would be if the ailment were taken away. Three great examples of this are the conditions of anxiety, depression and pain. If you have ever suffered one of these ailments, you know how different your quality of life is when a medication can take away the symptom. Depending on the person, sometimes it is more beneficial to clear the underlying links to the illness while on medication as they are fully present to do the work, and sometimes a person does better without medication as they feel their symptom so acutely that the work is more effective because of the acuteness of symptoms. We're all so different. There isn't a better or worse way to approach healing. It's purely based on what the patient resonates with best. Medications prescribed and expected to be used as a tool forever without looking at how your vibrational being is programmed remove an opportunity for you to get the most out of your life.

Many life experiences contribute to a person's symptoms. Our symptoms separate us not only from ourselves, but also from our lives. I'm offering you guidance to use your symptoms in an opposite way—to more deeply connect you to yourself. The exercise at the end of this chapter will teach you how to practice this.

With any illness, there often exists an endocrine imbalance that involves reproductive hormone levels as well as thyroid and adrenal imbalances. Blood sugar levels can be fluctuating, food allergies may be present, the immune system may be compromised where chronic viruses, bacteria or fungi may be interfering with cellular function. Although there are many possible causes to our internal imbalance, it's fascinating to see how these things have the ability to clear up on their own when self-love is our conviction. This brings such strength to the physical body that opportunistic situations can be eliminated. Opportunistic situations are those that, given the opportunity, will show their ugly heads. This term is usually applied to viruses, like herpes or shingles. The virus is always in the system, lying dormant, not causing any undue stress on your body most of the time. But when your immune system is compromised, the virus will surface. A few examples of things that can compromise our immune system are poor sleep, a high-sugar diet, caffeine, and unfortunate tragedies and losses.

Although in medicine, the definition of "opportunistic infection" applies to organisms in our system, I believe all illnesses are opportunistic. When the body is out of balance, our weak spots will be exposed. I see it all the time. If, however, our practice is to live in self-love and live in self-respect, we will maintain balance more effortlessly.

It's important to remember that self-love is a way of being but it does take practice. It does take awareness. It does take effort. It's a journey and it has its ups and downs just like all of life. These exercises, although simple, are powerful if you put them to practice daily. Practice means just that—practice. Do not expect to perfect them. I haven't met a person that has. It's also important to have fun with the practice.

These exercises are not just nice things to do. They are life-changing events as they affect the patterns within you that are currently keeping you stuck. You will begin to shift from surviving to living, from lack-of-ease to ease, from fear to love. Time and patience, not to mention self-love and joy, are essential factors in healing.

Now that you have an idea of just how your body holds your challenging emotions, let's talk a little bit about how to actually begin dissolving them into love.

Every single one of us will have challenging experiences in life. Self-honor creates the foundation for us to work within. Self-honor needs to be strong for this step to be effective. If you are having trouble with the first writing exercise or the second visualization exercise, keep practicing them before you move onto this step. This first step is about taking inventory. Once you've collected the data, you can begin shifting your habits to create more desired outcomes. You will be able to practice shifting your challenges into the very opportunities they were designed to be in the first place. It's important to remember that nothing happens by accident as you move into this next step. Believing this makes this next simple step easy. Simple and easy are two different things but we tend to confuse them. Simple means to stay focused on the little things that you can embrace. Easy to me means entering with ease. Believing that all things happen for a reason eases our experiences.

Simply choosing to believe that all the decisions that

you make are the correct ones for you gives you permission to live with joy.

> If you *could* give yourself permission to live with joy every moment of your life, would you?

If you could give yourself permission to live with joy each moment, you would, certainly. Why don't you? Why don't any of us? And when we choose to, what gets in our way? The answer is simple and I've mentioned it in an earlier chapter. We aren't taught to live this way. There is so much natural worrying—and as a child, you learn this by being around it. Worrying about being on time, having a clean home, doing or saying the right thing, making enough money, being thin enough—as a kid you would overhear these kinds of adult conversations all the time. Next time you're in a coffee shop or at a party, listen to the dialogues. These dialogues began to shape you as a child. Each of us has had unique childhood experiences—some more challenging than others. The thread that makes them all the same is that they are all opportunities. Our choices around and within them determine the outcome. And now, as adults, the same opportunities exist. The difference now is that we have the tools to interact with these opportunities in a more mature way.

To effectively be able to give yourself permission to live with joy each and every moment, you must first be able to observe how much respect you have for yourself and to strive to maintain a 100% level. In addition, you need to be able to be connected with your body deeply enough that you are able to get its feedback *at all times*. The purpose of the first two exercises in this book is to create your foundation. Give yourself permission to utilize them in this way.

Permission is an emotion of love. There are two balancing energies in and around us at all times, available for us to tap into at will. The two energies, as we have addressed earlier, are love and fear. Many, many authors speak of this delicate balance. Before you can freely choose which energy to function in, you must understand this basic truth. When you are happy, you are in a loving place. When you are feeling threatened, you are in a fearful place. These are obvious. Absolutely *any* emotion or feeling can be labeled as love or fear. Tenderness, compassion, joy, sharing, supporting, giving, receiving, and teaching are all examples of love. Jealousy, hatred, judgment, anger, low self-esteem, stealing, and lying are all examples of fear. Since we can only have one thought at a time, if our thought is of fear, it cannot be of love. It's simple. One thought at a time. One emotion at a time. Love or fear. Your choice.

Just as Wayne Dyer says, "If you feel good, you feel God." There is not a better example of love that I can think of. You may refer to your higher power as a different entity; no problem, it's all the same. Just replace the word God with what works for you. Please don't become offended; take your power back and just change the word to work for you. Being offended is another example of fear. I'm simply creating a reference point for you to connect with your belief system. One of my favorite teachers, Carolyn Myss, offers sound advice. She says "Choose to *never* take *anything* personally again." I guess this is one place where the word "never" does work.

In choosing to not take anything personally, you are giving yourself permission to maintain the space of love. Good self-esteem is reflected in a person who knows that part of life is making mistakes and that not everyone is going to like you—big deal! If you can accept these two beliefs, then you've eliminated about 95% of the difficulty in choosing love!

Let's go back to your childhood again. I'm sure you've heard conversations about what so and so did to me at the office or what so and so said about so and so. We get so involved in how everyone else feels and does things that we start doing the same thing without even realizing that we are giving our power away! We give our power away and we start to forget truly who we are. We end up judging others because it makes us feel better about ourselves—not in our heart, but in our mind, where the ego, our great protector of insecurity, lives. It has absolutely nothing to do with that other person; it's all to do with ourselves. It's like an invisible shield that protects us from our own insecurities. Weird, huh?

So, we've learned this, and it's no one's fault. All of us, including our parents, are always trying to do the best that we can. We simply weren't taught this level of doing our best. It's essential to teach and learn it now as a society because we are becoming so disconnected and less healthy. Again, I believe the epidemic of chronic disease to be the gift to reconnecting.

Choosing love then requires the knowledge that it is a choice. This next exercise changes lives.

Change Your Story

Think of a recent experience that was difficult for you. Close your eyes and play the whole thing in your mind as if you were watching a video of the whole scenario. Watch the details closely.

Remember where you were, who you were with, what the conversation was, etc. Watch this movie of you in your life as if it were happening again right now.

As you are watching the most challenging part of that experience, notice how your body feels. Notice clearly what your body is experiencing.

Whatever you notice, this is *where* your emotion is living in your body.

Take time now to silently be grateful to your body. Thank it directly for getting your attention so clearly and so immediately.

Now ask the question, "If love were my only option right now and I chose it, what would it do here?"; "If love could come into this situation and dissolve everything other that isn't love out of my body, what would happen here?"

Simply Notice.

The New You

Choose to use this exercise in every difficult situation.

It takes no time.

You don't have to share with anyone what you are doing.

If you find yourself in a difficult conversation, just take a deep breath and notice what your body is feeling.

Ask the question silently.

Deep breath again.

Allow all of your words and actions from this point forward to come from this place.

Your conversation just took a turn.

You're in your power and all is as it should be.

∞ Chapter 15 ∞

The Body

∫

Coming Home

We can now shift our study to the actual physical body, now that we have a good idea of the different energies that affect it. Your physical body is usually the first place in which you recognize an imbalance, even though it may not have started there.

Your body is made up of billions of cells. These cells are busy, busy, busy with more activity going on at all times than any of us can perceive. Hormones are shuttling things around, receptors are picking things up and opening doors into and out of cells, nutrients are constantly being metabolized, creating energy and waste at the same time. It is absolutely mind-boggling to visualize the ever-constant activity that occurs every second of your life without even a thought on your part. I see it visually like a billion little ants all running in different directions, but always working together in harmony.

Your physical body holds the space for your mind, emotions and spirit to animate itself in. Your body creates a boundary between you and the rest of the world. And that's about it. It is space. You are so much more than this. In fact, daily I share with people that the body is the smallest part of the actual self. It is a vehicle. If your vehicle is running smoothly and efficiently, you will accomplish more in life. More efficiency, more vitality, more joy because you will feel good physically.

Just as much as your mind, thoughts and emotions dictate the health of your body, so does your body dictate the health of your mind. It's a cycle that continuously feeds itself, without any beginning or end like a circle. If your body is well physically, your mind can be more at ease. If your body is achy, tired, your mind will reflect that as well. My mother-in-law has always been one of the funniest, kindest and most gentle people I know. As she ages and things hurt and she loses her energy to follow through physically on the things she wants to do mentally she becomes more and more cantankerous, outside of her wanting to be so. She complains about things that she never would have even noticed before. Perception is as deeply affected by the body as the body's health is affected by the mind. It's a circular and continuous relationship.

So how can we keep this vessel running like an efficient machine? First step is to love it regardless of where you are starting the tune-up from. I will share a personal story about this exact concept. About three months after my second baby was born I caught myself looking at my naked body in the mirror sideways. I pushed up the skin on my belly while sucking it in, I lifted my breasts and tucked my butt under . . . and the whole time thinking to myself, "Ugh, ugh, ugh!" I even had a frown on my face. Time stopped and I immediately let go of all the loose skin and thanked my body out loud for being a woman, for creating such beautiful children and for feeding them with my precious milk. My body never looked better than it did in that moment. How in the world can I teach what I do and not practice it? Oh, it hit me like a ton of bricks. Two weeks later, without making any conscious changes—I didn't change my diet or exercise—I had lost six pounds. Patients were commenting on how quickly I got my figure back after my babies.

You've probably had enough of the whole "body creation from the mind" thing. If you're bored with the whole topic, you don't understand its importance. I want you to be excited about it—not bored! So, if you are bored, go back and re-read it all and when you get here, it will be more fun. This part of healing is the part of medicine that is missing. I'm not talking about the need for psychotherapy. I'm talking about awareness of your life, honor of yourself, love of your choices and manifestation of health. Everything we've talked about until now is the *foundation*. Just like my yoga teacher, Cintra Brown, would always say, "You would never build a house on sand."

This brings us back to your temple, your vessel, your physical world. Your lifestyle, or style of living, creates a body that is either balanced or unbalanced. You know right now which one is true for you. Lifestyle consists of your dietary practices, exercise regimens, and stress levels—which include your career and your relationships. Your medical and inherited conditions will both be reflective of and contributory to your lifestyle. Let's have fun exploring your body through understanding your lifestyle.

Your Body in Your Life

Close your eyes and scan your body with this question—"What does it feel like to be me in my body right now?"

Get to know what your body feels in this moment.

Now, play a video of a typical day in your mind. Visualize with detail each event that occurs from the moment you wake up until the time you go to bed.

Literally watch yourself live a typical day.

Notice the decisions you make each day on how to spend your time.

As you're watching, notice how your body feels through all the different experiences. Notice if your body feels different at work than it does at home.

Notice how your lifestyle feels in your body.

If you notice discomfort at specific times, this is your body telling you that the particular event isn't supportive of optimal health and will require a little more attention.

Journal what you experienced.

∞ Chapter 16 ∞

The Body

∫

Nurture Yourself

The body's functioning ability and efficiency depends on vital nutrients. With them, it absorbs, eliminates, metabolizes, and communicates perfectly. Without them, the cells have their own way of letting you know—you get symptoms! If you have symptoms, of any kind, your body is simply asking for something. Let's start by giving it life-sustaining nutrients.

The body's ability to incorporate nutrients into the system in order to build our cells, neurotransmitters, hormones, bones, et cetera, depends on optimal nutrition, hydration, elimination, exercise and rest. For this chapter, we'll focus on nutrition. An important thing to note here, before we get deeper into the subject, is that it often takes years of poor nutrition before symptoms appear. What's more important to point out is that people often blame their symptoms on just about anything else, not their lifestyle. It takes education about how nutrition impacts our cells first (which is usually not immediately noticeable), body systems next (which start to get our attention) and finally overall health—or lack of it—which is what brings us to the doctor. This book will briefly skim the necessary ideas about how to begin thinking about nutrition.

Optimal nutrition is tricky for several reasons. The produce section of a general grocery store is compromised due to over-cultivation of the soil rendering the foods nutrient-deficient by nature. In packaged foods, there are preservatives, additives, colors and binders necessary to keep the food from spoiling quickly and also to make it look pretty. Unfortunately, the "better-tasting" foods that people enjoy are laden with nutrient-deficient, calorie-dense ingredients. Processed foods are cheaper than unadulterated foods, as their shelf lives are longer and they are made in massive quantities. Isn't it cheaper to get a Coke instead of bottled water when you're eating lunch out?

In addition to the differences in food qualities available, there are also a lot of opinions when it comes to nutrition. If there were a diet that worked well to keep us all healthy with lots of robust energy and kept us all at our ideal weights with minimal health risk factors, there would only be one diet, right? There are more books on nutrition than any of us would ever really have any need of. And many people own more nutrition and diet books than they would like to admit. Each new diet book that comes out seems to be *the* book until the next one comes out, and you are still the same weight and have the same low amount of energy, and you're still going to the doctor and receiving the same findings of high cholesterol, high blood pressure, fatigue, et cetera, and possibly a higher weight than last year.

So, what's on the shelf? The low fat diets have gratefully run out of fashion but the high protein diets unfortunately are strongly in vogue right now. These diets tend to be the "miracle" diets for most as rapid weight loss occurs initially. Once the success starts to wane, people generally give up and gain the weight back and then some. This is due to the hormonal imbalances that occur with long term exposure to high protein diets. You end up with organ system challenges that produce extreme stress on the body and ultimately end up with glandular problems that can then take years to "fix."

Why, I ask you, is more than 60% of the population overweight if the diet books that are available are effective? We have the knowledge—just pick up a book, right? Wrong.

One important aspect of nutrition that I begin sharing with my patients is, "It's not what you're eating that is the problem. It's *why* you're eating what you're eating." Do you think Dr. Phil has any training in nutrition? He probably does now, but is he a nutritionist? No—he's a psychologist! And he's probably got the most successful weight loss book on the market! The top two reasons why I feel people struggle with weight issues (which begins the degradation of the body and leads to chronic ailments) is #1—the lack of knowledge and #2—too much stress to do anything about it.

Since my intent is not to make this a weight loss book, allow me to refer you to the best nutritional book available today called *The Program*, by Diana Schwarzbein. Her motto is "You must be healthy to lose weight, not lose weight to be healthy." I'll admit that before I started studying with her I made mistakes with recommending high protein diets to my patients. My saving grace was that I also insisted on lots of fresh vegetables with the high protein.

In general now, I'll present to you where I start when I speak of nutritional healing to patients. As I present my principles of nutrition to you, remember—your motivations are just as important as your knowledge. Knowledge is power, motivation is action. The most exciting aspect of the very first weight loss program at our clinic was the consistency of praise about all of the things that they *gained* as they *lost* weight. Higher energy levels, clearer thinking, better sleep, a decrease in medication use—some people even decided to make career moves to support this new phase of life they had stepped into. None of them thought a weight loss program would offer all of that. In my opinion, if it doesn't, it will only be temporary success. I recognize now that if the support doesn't continue, the success will also be temporary. Until we are each individually strong in our mind-body-spirit being, we access strength in being accountable to something *outside* of ourselves rather than *to* ourselves. This takes breaking patterns that have been programmed in our thoughts and emotions for years and years.

Nutrition is a lifestyle, not a fad. Healing programs need to continue on long enough for the participants to have adapted a shift in their natural rhythm of living life to one that exhibits natural self-love and self-honor. This new rhythm has to be a great enough priority in their lives for them to continue self-care—as a lifestyle.

I refer to several nutrition books in my practice so that

people can have a reference point. I never recommend, however, any single book to be used alone. *The Program* as mentioned above is primary. A complementary book that I also respect is Dr. D'Adamo's , *Eat Right for Your Type*. This book gives people a general idea about which particular foods are better or worse for their bodies. Not only do I respect the research behind the program that identifies why there are differing responses to food based on our blood type, I clinically observe pretty quick results when patients shift their foods for their blood type. If my patients aren't inclined to pick up the book, I'll offer food allergy testing.

The higher protein books that I used to recommend like Barry Sears's book called *The Zone* and the *Atkins Diet* and *Protein Power* by Eades, and now *The South Beach Diet*—all are pretty similar. My absolute concern that I have with these diets is that quality of proteins is rarely discussed and that carbohydrates get a really bad name. The quality of carbohydrates is really what people need to know, and Anne Louise Gittleman does a great job with this in her book *The Fat Flush*. I do like Suzanne Somers's book called *Somersize*; however, I am not a proponent at all of artificial sweeteners. If you use her wisdom, just replace all the artificial sweeteners with the sweet, no-calorie herb—very safe to be taken orally—called *stevia*.

Then there's Dr. Crook, who has popularized the Candida Diet, high in protein and complex carbohydrates. I refer to his writing frequently for the educational piece about the organism candida since it is such a chronic condition, but I use *The Program* as the backbone of any program. Candida is a condition that thrives on sugar. Candida is a fungus, a yeast that is a necessary part of the natural digestive tract. When it becomes imbalanced compared to other natural organisms in the body, we get in trouble. It becomes unbalanced with specific exposures like antibiotics, birth control pills, steroids and sugar.

I refer to various educational materials because people need education and are hoping for expertise that is correct for optimal body metabolism and health management. The nutritional guidance I offer at my clinic is one that statistically reduces symptoms and risk factors that would otherwise contribute to an early demise or worse—a poor quality of a long life.

This program includes dietary assistance as well as a stress management system and exercise program. The reason that this program is so successful is because it breaks the rhythm that you are engaged in now that is not working for you. The tools are simple, and you have regular check-in points at which we evaluate numerous aspects of your health: your cell membrane integrity, the electrical conduction between cells, your nutrition versus waste balance, your lean body mass to fat ratio, and hydration status. Patients get motivated by witnessing their first reading, which may indicate toxicity at the level of the cell, or a high fat mass compared to lean mass or simply a state of dehydration that prevents anything from moving or shifting in your body. This is the motivational beginning. Then, based on your results, a very specific plan is designed with you that actually encourages "real" carbohydrates, with the inclusion of "healthy" grain carbohydrates, combined with healthy proteins and an emphasis on "good" fat. Some patients eat away from home as a rule, and can follow this plan with ease; the joy comes in the retesting. As the program continues, patients shift their goals because they are feeling better and feeling younger and healthier and have a newly discovered optimism. I am grateful to see my patients making themselves worthy enough to pay attention to themselves and to feel a sense of ease about themselves that wasn't there initially. My biggest joy is when patients increase their expectation of health! Something changes. People live with a newly-found confidence. It's beautiful. There is a felt balance in life.

Balance is what it's all about. Since the body metabolizes food efficiently within two to three hours, we should be eating that frequently. If you have a cup of coffee in the morning and don't eat again until dinner—does that sound balanced? Many people live this way, believe it or not. I joke with my patients and say that I believe we are evolving into robots. People are so dehydrated and eat such adulterated foods, if they make time for it, and we just keep going— with fatigue and memory loss and weight gain, but we keep going. Frequency is the first step to nutritional balancing—eat something every three hours. Once this occurs we'll get to what's *optimal* to eat every three hours. First adopt the rhythm. If you are able to do this, this addresses the beginning of balancing your stress hormones in two ways; through both food (frequency) and the choice to slow down enough to make it happen.

What are we eating at these frequent intervals? You have to think about breakfast, lunch, dinner and snacks between each meal and at bedtime. For the meals, visualize a plate and on it build a meal around a protein. Pick your protein first. This should be the size and thickness of about ¼ to ½ of your palm. Now pick your carbohydrate or starch or fruit next. This should be about the same size of your protein. Three times the size of your palm should be vegetables—the majority of your plate. Then, become open to learning about grains like quinoa, kamut, spelt, and millet, consider whole rice instead of white, and please garnish with some sort of fat. Use oil as your dressing, such as avocado, sesame, olive or flaxseed oil blend on vegetables and salads. Fat from organic whole butter for garnish and nut butters like almond, sesame and cashew are also encouraged. Your body needs fat. Every cell in your body has a cell wall around it. These cell walls are made up of fat—a bi-lipid (two fats facing each other) membrane. The more unsaturated the fat, the better, unless of course you're frying something, in which case you'll be best off using coconut oil. Since the inception of fat-free diets, obesity has exponentially increased. I'm sure there are other contributing factors, but fat-free diets haven't helped obesity to decline. NOR HAVE HIGH PROTEIN DIETS!

Snacks between meals don't have to be anything fancy. Consider a handful of almonds with a half piece of fruit or handful of berries, yogurt, celery stuffed with nut butter, a hard-boiled egg, perhaps, or leftover slices of chicken dipped in a dressing of sorts, or rolled up in lettuce leaves. Have fun and be creative.

What I'm describing requires planning. Boy, do I feel it if I haven't shopped and prepared for the week. Then I'm calling restaurants and ordering take-out each night that week. Sometimes this happens, and when it does, we've got to go with it and pray extra hard over the food and love it. Most importantly, preparation is the key. Convenience stores and drive-thrus won't support your endeavors to eat well.

Sometimes I think people believe that anything in a package with a 5-year shelf life will also preserve their body!

I mentioned dehydration. We should be drinking half of our body weight in ounces of water per day if you're not active, more if you are. So, if you weigh 150 pounds, you should be drinking 75 ounces of water per day. If you drink caffeine, that good old dehydrating-yet-stimulating substance, you must drink two glasses of water of equal size to your caffeinated beverage just to get up to a baseline of hydration. Let's say that you drink a six-ounce cup of coffee each morning and a twelve-ounce glass of iced tea at lunch. You must drink 2 six-ounce cups of water to cover the coffee and 2 twelve-ounce glasses of water to cover your tea, equaling 36 ounces of water just to catch up! The same exact rule applies to alcohol intake. We haven't mentioned cleaning your liver out from all these chemicals, we're just talking hydration. So many people believe that their coffee or tea or soda is hydrating them. How many people like a nice cold beer after working in the yard all day? Lots.

The tool that helps most of us break patterns of a poor diet is to write it down. Preferably you are doing this in the beginning of the week as you are planning your meals and shopping lists. If you have been this organized, reflect back to the day's plan each night to see how well you did. If you're still shooting from the hip and choosing a meal at a time, take time each night before you go to bed, think back on your day and write down everything you ate and drank. It's good to have a mirror to look into to reflect back to you what you are doing. Bad habits are easier to fall into if we're not paying attention. If we don't stop to look at our habits, we could easily ignore them and move on, pretending that it never happened. If we do this time and time again, eating poorly becomes unconscious suicide.

Keeping a diet ledger doesn't have to be anything fancy. You can use a spiral pad if you like. I'll share the type of weekly planner that I like to use. I prepare my entire week's menu on the weekend. I organize my recipes and know ahead of time if I need to stop for fresh produce. I'll prepare my meats ahead of time with seasonings and vacuum-seal them in the freezer. I'll even flash-freeze vegetables for the freezer if the week is full and time is short. Crockpots are also a great tool for busy moms, with better and better cookbooks available on this subject like *Not Your Mother's Slow Cooker Cookbook* by Beth Hensperger. Whatever helps you to be more efficient in your menu planning, use it. Being prepared is the *most important aspect of eating well!*

Recently, a book has been published called *The Hidden Messages in Water*, by Masaru Emoto. This is a masterpiece. The author spent countless years with a photographer mastering the photographing of a crystal of water. Once perfected, he would repeatedly demonstrate how much our thoughts affect water crystals in a glass of water. When groups of people got together and focused thoughts of love towards a glass of water, the crystals would look like diamonds with breathtaking crystalline beauty. When, on the other hand, thoughts of hatred were delivered to the water, the crystals either shattered or were left with black holes in the center and distorted edges. He collected water from different parts of the world and displayed how vastly different earth energy is in the various parts of the world. Musical vibration was also studied. Symphonies were compared to punk rock, with expected results.

If water *outside* of the body is so influenced by our thoughts, what effect do you think that our thoughts have over the water *inside* of our body? Our bodies are on average 70% water. Should it be any surprise that our thoughts have a powerful effect over the health of our bodies?

So, not only is hydration essential, it carries the harmonious or disharmonious connection of each cell to each other. Marvelous work. With each sip of water, silently bless yourself.

Weekly Food Planner

		Protein	Vegetable	Grain or Starchy Vegetable	Fruit	Fat
Monday	Breakfast					
	Snack					
	Lunch					
	Snack					
	Dinner					
	Snack					
Tuesday	Breakfast					
	Snack					
	Lunch					
	Snack					
	Dinner					
	Snack					
Wednesday	Breakfast					
	Snack					
	Lunch					
	Snack					
	Dinner					
	Snack					
Thursday	Breakfast					
	Snack					
	Lunch					
	Snack					
	Dinner					
	Snack					
Friday	Breakfast					
	Snack					
	Lunch					
	Snack					
	Dinner					
	Snack					
Saturday	Breakfast					
	Snack					
	Lunch					
	Snack					
	Dinner					
	Snack					
Sunday	Breakfast					
	Snack					
	Lunch					
	Snack					
	Dinner					
	Snack					

∞ Chapter 17 ∞

The Body

∫

Letting Go

This chapter isn't about letting go of stress; rather, it's about letting go of waste. If we are taking food into our body several times per day, we should be eliminating several times per day. The very reason you are surprised at that statement is the reason that I'm reserving an entire chapter for it.

"Poop" is as common a word as "baseball" in our family. For most, it is a private experience never shared with others. I'm not only comfortable with discussing it with my family and my patients, but it also gives me great joy when optimal experiences are described. Patients will describe the "normal for me" poop, which quite frequently is not the "normal for health" poop. Whenever my kids are cranky I look for one of the three triggers: (1) they're hungry, (2) they didn't get enough sleep or, (3) they need to poop. This is just another example of how our body health affects our emotions.

There is a statement I say just about every day in my practice. This belief guides me in treating each and every patient, regardless of what they came in for. This is it:

> Your body is as healthy as its ability to eliminate waste.

If you take in food, you should be eliminating waste. To have a metabolism means that you are constantly creating waste. No work is done in the body that doesn't create waste products. I'm not just talking about your bowel movements. I'm talking about each cell of your body. To do *anything*, the cell requires fuel and creates waste. If waste accumulates around your cells or organs or glands, the cell, organ or gland starts to function less optimally. It congests the system. I believe that we accumulate waste into our weak spots. If your cells were functioning optimally, if there were proper nutrition to and waste flow away from each cell, there would be no expression of an imbalance.

You may accumulate waste into a headache, or into joint pain or into congestion and allergies or into depression . . . whatever your symptoms, this is where your weak spot is. So, each diagnosis simply tells me how that person is accumulating waste. If there is a nutrient lacking or if there isn't enough water to carry waste away, cellular elimination is backed up and the cell's job is affected. Then the cells start communicating to you through inflammation or fatigue or irritability—whatever your first symptom of lack-of-ease in your body is—and hopefully you can hear their message.

So, if a person comes in with headaches, the first thing I want to know about their physical body is how they're eliminating. Of course patterns of elimination are a reflection of what people eat, what they drink, what compromises have occurred to their intestines and liver from medication exposures, surgeries, et cetera. Many times, my first goal with patients is for them to have at least one bowel movement daily.

If a woman desires bio-identical hormone replacement therapy, I want to know how she's eliminating for several reasons. The liver is the main waste elimination organ. It not only detoxifies the body, it must break down everything that we take into the body from food to herbs and medications. If its job is compromised at all, utilization of nutrients and medications will be much less efficient. In addition, a compromised liver doesn't clean the body efficiently, creating this backup of waste. Think of your liver like a vacuum bag. You must empty the bag to keep cleaning after it is full, right? This is the same idea of a detoxification or a cleansing, which is becoming more and more popular. If you think of your liver now as a sponge, a cleansing squeezes out the sponge so all the dirty water leaves. I will mention briefly that if you choose to do a detoxification program, as the layers of physical waste shift out of the body, so do the emotional patterns that have become attached to that waste. This is a good time to journal and to expect lots of movement, not just from your bowels but from the emotional you. Sometimes this is the reason that I begin treating a person through a detoxification program—to clear out emotions and toxins that may cloud the view of what the body-mind-spirit specifically need once the dust clears out. Sometimes the cleanse is the only guidance the person needed.

One of the liver's main tasks is to conjugate and eliminate hormones in our body. This is why, if I have a woman with severe PMS or endometriosis or infertility, I begin by cleaning out the liver. This is essential. There are globulins in the liver. Their job is to bind hormones for use in the body. If these are compromised, we have hormonal changes. Our success rate in treating hormone-related conditions, including infertility, with simply cleansing and supporting the liver is astronomical—and it's a lot of fun. One of the reasons it's so fun is because it's so simple. Moreover, not only is the woman grateful for her symptom resolution, she is much healthier overall, and other things that we weren't even treating also improve. Lastly, women are happier with a clean liver. The main emotion of a congested liver is irritability. This definition comes from traditional Chinese medicine. We may get more irritable in the cleansing process, but as things move out and clear, there is a personality shift towards peace, ease and grace. My office staff likes when that happens.

In addition to the liver, the intestines contribute much to our ability to eliminate waste. They not only carry the waste out, but they will also reabsorb toxins into the body that further challenge the overall functioning of the cells of the body, including liver detoxification again. The reabsorbed toxins tend to be even more harsh on the system than they were on the first go-around.

Some women going through menopause want to transition without the use of any hormone therapy. Most of the focus on these women will be on cleansing the liver and intestines, in addition to supporting the adrenal glands, and whatever else shows up for the particular patient. So many women notice that a simple sip of wine can cause immediate hot flashes or a bad night's sleep. This is the liver correlation. In the society that we live in with all the things that compromise our systems from polluted air to adulterated food to poor sleep, natural menopause can become a full time job. It is possible, and it is beautiful to watch. If, on the other hand, a woman desires bioidentical hormone therapy, I know that the hormones will be giving more work to her liver. Even a substance that may be more beneficial to have than to not have still requires the liver to do more work.

You're as healthy as your body's ability to eliminate waste. What exactly influences our waste elimination? Here are the principles, in no specific order of importance—*they're all equally important*. You already know about optimal fluid intake. Fiber requirement is a simple fact at 30-35 grams daily, and grossly underachieved in our society. I described earlier—very broadly—optimal nutrition as a place to start. I do lab testing for nutrient levels on patients to diagnose individual deficiencies. This is very helpful in the clinical setting to speed up the healing process; remember that if the cells have optimal nutrition, they will function more efficiently.

Exercise itself aids elimination significantly by increasing circulation to and away from each cell. At the same time, exercise also increases the metabolism of each cell, thereby creating more waste. If your nutrition and fluid intakes are optimal, then there will be a net increase in waste elimination with exercise.

Keys to Enhance Elimination

Optimal Hydration
Half your body weight in ounces of water per day, minimum.
Increase for:
increased physical activity
caffeinated beverages
high-salt and -sugar foods
processed foods

Optimal fiber
30-35 grams of fiber daily.

Optimal Nutrition
Add specific extra nutritional support for your individual biochemistry.

Optimal exercise
Increases muscle tone of your intestines as well as abdominal muscles.

Optimal Stress Management
Allows cells of body, especially bowels, to relax and function optimally.

∞ Chapter 18 ∞

The Body

∫

Movement

Now that we have nutrients in our body, and hopefully optimal ones to build up the body cells from neurotransmitters to hormones to our skeletal, nervous, and glandular systems, let's begin thinking of moving them through us with more than just water.

I'd like to use the word "movement" instead of "exercise" because it's much more friendly to most people who aren't used to the concept of exercise as part of their daily routine. I personally don't think of optimal exercise as going to the gym and hitting it so hard that you sweat half your body water out and kick up your adrenaline to get the "high" that so many athletes speak of. As we age, we need more resistance and stretching than stimulating exercise. Examples of resistance exercises are weight training mat exercises, strengthening yoga, Pilates—the idea being that your heart rate is not elevated higher than 90 beats per minute for longer than a few minutes and recovers to below 90 before you begin your next exercise. In Diana Schwarzbein's book, *The Program* she states that, "The truth is that over doing cardiovascular or stimulating exercise is bad for your heart and your metabolism because it breaks you down, especially after the age of 35-40 when you are entering the normal aging phase of your life. The more you do of these types of exercise, the faster you will age and the more heart attacks you can expect, and the only type of weight loss you will "successfully" achieve is the loss of lean body tissues that include organs, bones, and muscle as well as your fat stores." She goes on to say that, "on average, a Tibetan Monk who does yoga and meditates lives longer and has less heart disease than an American athlete who is involved in some type of running sport."

I couldn't agree with her more. While many of us "over-exercise", an equal to greater number of us "under-exercise". Walking leisurely and light stretching enhance our circulation which brings nutrients to and waste away from the cells much more than sitting idle behind a computer does. If you have a sitting job, it's important to stand and stretch every so often to open the channels of circulation and nerve conduction. This is a good way to begin thinking of movement if it's not part of your vocabulary yet.

Notice how children play on the playground. One of the playgrounds we frequent has lots of sand under all of the play areas and water features to run through. Notice how much the children move their bodies. Notice how they don't groan when they bend down to pick up a shovel from the sand and how they run form swing to slide to monkey bars—smiling and laughing. Most moms and dads will say, "Boy those kids just crashed tonight after playing all day."

Notice also how kids get grouchy and moody when they haven't done much with their physical bodies during the day—perhaps a rainy day or a Game-cube day, God for bid. Those Game-Cubes and X-Boxes are something we as parents need to accept on some level—with minimal time exposure to them. Otherwise, as I stated previously, all the excitement and energy enters through the thumbs and gets trapped in the little bodies. Parents will make very different statements regarding their kids on those less active days. It's as clear as when a kid is hungry or not.

My point here is that if we move our bodies (like kids do), we sleep better (like kids do) and we're happier (like kids are). A lot of times movement just takes getting into the habit. I can certainly appreciate the reality of living a busy life and not having time. Remember that healing requires you making time for you. It doesn't have to be much—stretch your body every few hours for a few minutes. Walk leisurely with loved ones in the evening as the sun sets. Find ways for movement to be not only fun but something you actually look forward to. You'll sleep better, live happier and minimize the degenerative diseases of aging.

∞ *Chapter 19* ∞

The Body

∫

Your Shock Absorbers

Life has changed a lot over the past forty years. Lifestyles are so different compared to what they were when our parents were parents. Rarely was there the need for a two-income household. As kids, we walked and rode our bikes everywhere and played in the woods with the other neighborhood kids, never wondering if a stranger was going to show up and kidnap us or hurt us. Commercials were suitable for viewing by all audiences, and ADD wasn't a household diagnosis.

We're here now in the 21st century, enjoying the luxuries of fast-paced living. There seems to be one Starbucks for every 20 homes in any given neighborhood. Thank goodness, for where else would I get my quick caffeine fix on my way home from work so I can get the million and one things that need doing done before dawn the next day?

But there's balance. You can go to any convenience store and buy an ice tea or fruit drink with Ginseng in it. Ginseng, known as an adrenal tonifier, balances the over-secretion of adrenaline, our get-up-and-go hormone. It kind of nurtures those tiny little adrenal glands that buffer stress all day long for you. We just push, push, push, all day long and when we feel like we can't keep going, we'll consume an adrenaline-like substance like caffeine to give the body a false sense that it can keep going. Poor sleep is a symptom of and a contributor to adrenal fatigue. The same thing goes for our inability to handle stress or to make good choices for ourselves.

When I describe the need for people to spend time breathing, meditating, praying, journaling, taking relaxing baths, walking, reading, being creative—even just taking a supplement twice a day—people cannot find time! We have got to find time to come home to ourselves. Just like the challenged liver manifesting irritability, challenged adrenal glands manifest lack of safety. This is why anxiety is an expression of adrenal imbalance. You absolutely cannot feel safe, peaceful, and relaxed if you're stressed. They are polar opposites.

Not only do your adrenals have to start kicking up the action to meet the demands on the body due to stress, every other cell of the body responds as well. Although the body is made up of different systems, you are an entire system. When one part of you suffers or needs more support to do its job well, the other cells are aware of this and shift to accommodate. Your body is like communities within communities, all trying to help each other out. Regardless of your symptoms, your whole body pays the price by adapting and accommodating. You can see this on a very simple level if you consider the nutrient L-Glutamine. This is an amino acid that has three very distinct roles in the body. One is in the gut, another in the brain and the third in the adrenal glands. If your adrenal glands need more fuel to keep up with the demand it will beg, borrow and steal fuel from the other body parts. Could this possibly be why we see so many digestive complaints and failing memories? Stress affects the whole body. It comes up with 95% of my patients. We all think we "can handle it." Why do we want to, and for how long do we want to go on trying? Until our bodies break down and say, "No more?"

What's really a challenge is when people sign up for stress management classes and stress out to get there on time and then find a way to focus on all the things they *should* be doing instead. We've all been there and it's no picnic. There's lots of research supporting the truth that stress is cumulative. Therefore, taking a break in the middle of a stressful situation, instead of grinding through, will interrupt the snowballing effect, even if it's for a short time. The Europeans have it down. Two hours in the middle of the day—everything is closed, people go home, have a siesta, or whatever they desire.

Reflect back on the exercise of asking, "If love was my only option, what would it do here?" This puts a pause in the middle of a stressful event. You break the accumulation right there. Stress and fear are synonymous. Choose love and you've interrupted that snowballing out-of-control emotion. It takes time to work with these tools because we are in such set habits. With practice however, we really do break patterns. If your pattern is one of stress, you need to first recognize it and then start to find ways to interrupt it and possibly put a 180 on it. Be patient and loving to yourself in the meantime; it does take time. Recognize it, though. Be aware of how your whole body pays the price. Although it may not be to the point of your having Chronic Fatigue Syndrome, you don't want to wait for that to happen to do something about it.

What's interesting to me is how many people don't even recognize their stress level. I was one of them. Twice in the past three years I sought out counseling because I wasn't happy. My first counselor moved. My second counselor told me the exact same thing as the first one—I was too busy. The first counselor flat out said that if I didn't slow down, not only would I burn out and lose my career, I would also lose my relationship. The second pointed out that the only alone time I had was driving back and forth to work and even then I was studying audiotapes of one of my inspirational teachers. I understand the challenges involved in slowing down. At first it felt like I needed to release some of my passions. I realize now that I can embrace so many more passions that I didn't even know that I had.

Slowing down requires releasing some fears. What will you lose if you slow down? Perhaps it would be easier to ponder: what are you gaining from being so busy? I used to believe that being busy was a form of success. I realize now that having the courage to slow down is a greater symbol of success. Without chaos we are by nature more successful—not to mention healthier and happier.

One of my patients was a very successful young man, working long, hard hours, making lots of money. He told me that he would complain about the long days and physical work, and remembered wishing that he didn't have to work so hard to make a living. He had these thoughts every night. Within the next few months of his having these ideas, he was diagnosed with fibromyalgia and chronic fatigue syndrome. He was on disability until he retired and then came to me for help because he was suicidal.

Pause and Breathe

Take a moment to rest your body into a comfortable position.

Close your eyes. For the next few moments, just notice your breath.

Allow the breath its natural rhythm without forcing it or judging it—simply observe.

The breath occurs effortlessly without conscious control. It is the foundation of the rhythm within your body.

By noticing your chest rising and falling gently, you can become as relaxed as if you were sitting in front of an ocean, watching the waves breaking on the shoreline.

Notice the natural pause that exists between exhaling and inhaling.

If thoughts enter your mind, notice them and choose to let them go.

Reconnect to the movement of your breath.

Before you complete this time away from chaos, affirm to yourself that all is as it should be and all is well.

∞ Chapter 20 ∞

The Body

∫

Relationships

When I first started in practice I did a lot of acupuncture. At that time, I predominantly treated women. My success rate at treating ailments was pretty good, but I had a higher number of women who, after their series of treatments, were getting divorced.

Acupuncture brings balance to the body as it evens out the flow of energy through the meridians that connect and harmonize all of the systems of the body. I suppose the correlation between the acupuncture and the divorces was one of creating balance.

Our relationships are pivotal to our happiness. In relationship, we mirror each other. In a loving space, the mirror is one of self-honor and value. In a non-loving space, the mirror can be dreadful. Our mirrors and conversations are shaping us and molding us daily. If you are happier and healthier *because* of your relationships, congratulations, and enjoy! If you are happy and healthy *in spite* of your relationship, pay attention. If you are sad and sick because of your relationship, say goodbye!

Think about the law of attraction. If you are at odds most of the time with your partner, notice how the energy is keeping it together. If there is a way for you to choose to shift your energy to self-honor, you can do so. This would mean focusing only on what you love about your partner and your relationship to your partner. What you focus on will grow stronger. If you are focusing on what you dislike or what hurts, your focus brings more of that energy to the relationship and the cycle will never be broken. Both partners need to commit to this. If this takes too much work, or if you find very little positive things to focus on, you can access a third party to help with your communication, or you could simply exit the relationship. The problem with simply exiting is that you may never know your potential together. If you've had an objective, well-trained therapist work with you and you're still at odds, notice how you are benefiting from the relationship. If you don't choose to exit, and you choose instead to take responsibility and participate within the relationship the way you want to be treated, your partner will need to mirror this or the relationship will naturally lose the magnetism that keeps it together.

You can see how two people sharing in tenderness and passion and honor maintain their energy magnetism. You can probably see how two people sharing in criticisms and insults maintain their energy magnetism. Now see one person choosing to move into a place of love for self and the second not quite maturing to this level. Where's the magnetism? The second person will either need to learn how to share in that level of energy, or he or she will be phased out of the relationship. It is natural.

Mirror, Mirror on the Wall

The best way to discover if your relationship is supportive is to take time to write down your "wants" list. Write down everything you really want in a relationship. Write this list without thinking of your current relationship. This is not a list about what you are experiencing in your current relationship, this is a list about you. Even if you've been married for 50 years, come into yourself and notice what is important to you in a loving relationship.

Now go back over the list and circle anything that is an absolute need—that without which you would not feel deeply satisfied and honored as a partner. The things you do not circle are nice things that you would like but the loss of which would not cause you much distress.

If you are in a relationship, notice how many of your circled items are being met and how many are not. You will know by looking at it if your self esteem is being suppressed in your relationship.

If you are not in a relationship, you now have more joy knowing what you will not sacrifice when you choose your next partner.

∞ Chapter 21 ∞

The Spirit

∫

Surrender

The spirit body is the body of unconditional love. It is the energy that holds the space for the journey to unfold. It is always a net that we can go back to—to express, understand, and surrender to.

The word surrender brings up a lot of curiosity. The solar plexus is the part of the body that holds the stomach and intestines. This is the physical place where we carry our issues of control. Stomach issues like heartburn, bloating, irritable bowel syndrome—anything causing the stomach to be symptomatic—reflect an issue of control. Learning to let go opens the door to healing the physical stomach. Letting go is symbolically reflected in optimal bowel patterns of elimination. Holding on with an inability to let things go effortlessly can also manifest in an irritated, painful lining. The very word "irritated" indicates a need to learn to let go on some level. If you knew how, you would not choose to be irritated, right? We choose every experience. When we blame things outside of ourselves for our irritation, we are choosing to not take responsibility. In every moment we do have a choice. Surrendering to this truth gives you the highest level of control. Hence, you will no longer have control issues, and you will be effortlessly living in surrender.

If you weren't curious about surrender before reading that paragraph, hopefully you are now. Synonyms of surrender are "give in," "give up," and "submit." They don't sound too inviting, do they? But what if you used them in reference to your higher power? What if you gave in to your higher power, which is the symbol of unconditional love and acceptance of all things, completely? Would that be so bad? Doesn't it allow you the potential to let go of anything that is distracting from your higher power and completely submit to it as your guidance? This means that you are not submitting to fear, jealousy, judgment, and anger, to name a few. You choose instead to surrender to your higher power. Your higher power represents unconditional love.

I feel that I am the most powerful, the most at ease, and the most peaceful when I am able to totally and completely surrender to God. I connect with my potential to love in the deepest possible way. Daily, however, we are distracted by typical life stuff. Our energy is so strongly affected by life stuff—and it should be. Life stuff is you and me and our pets and our co-workers and the driver in the next lane and the checkout person at your neighborhood grocery store. We are all encased in these bodies that carry our unique expression of our higher power. So not only are we affected by the presence of each, we are affected by the choices each of us makes to live in love or to live in fear.

You can pick up a phone and call someone halfway around the Earth. Your energy is connected through the phone lines. You cannot see the energy but you can feel it because you can hear the words of your friend who may be looking at the sun while you're looking at the moon! When you are near certain people you may feel one way and totally differently with other people. Think back to when you were, perhaps, in school and switched classes. Each class was entirely different—the information (energy), the people in the class (energy), the location of the class (energy)…you cannot see it but you can feel it. Imagine yourself walking into a room where people just found out that a relative has died—does that feel different than when you walk into the room where a baby was just born? Of course.

How, then, do we surrender to our higher power with all the distractions going on around us all the time? That's just it. They are distractions. Each distraction that feels challenging is just another opportunity to connect more deeply to your higher power, to your potential to love—regardless of how difficult or easy the challenge itself is. The challenges are symbols of opportunity, just as your physical body is a symbol or manifestation of the total you—your mind, lifestyle, and your spirit. The first step in surrender is Gratitude.

The next exercise I'm offering you was taught to me at a seminar put on by Carolyn Myss. With hundreds of people in one room, Carolyn had a co-worker present this exercise to the group with great impact. Although a personal experience done in a group could typically be intimidating, it was absolutely perfect, as she had set the stage for everyone to be in a place of surrender to what is. I hope that your reading of this exercise brings to you as much healing as the directed words brought to me and the hundreds of other people in the group.

Turning the Fragmented You into the Integrated You

Close your eyes and center yourself within.

Once completely comfortable, welcome into your awareness an image of someone you have unhealed energy with.

Willingly welcome this person so clearly that you can feel their energy right there with you.

Now, as you see this person, notice that this person is nothing but an angel in a physical body—who was delivered directly to you on purpose.

The purpose of this angel in your life is to offer you an opportunity that no one else could offer to you.

The opportunity you are receiving is the practice of remaining in your space of unconditional love regardless of life's challenges. You get to practice raising your vibration to a lighter and lighter space, which is the space of unconditional love, regardless of the pain this person may have seemingly brought into your life.

Before you end your visualization, thank this person silently for the gift that they brought to you.

You may need to repeat this exercise several times before you feel free.

∞ Chapter 22 ∞

The Spirit

$$\int$$

Gratitude

Each part of this book is an extension of the others or a complement to the others. This is exactly the way I appreciate the body and the healing process. Each part, be it physical, emotional, or spiritual, is an extension of and a complement to the others. Within this system exists a rhythm. You have an observed rhythm of your day, starting with waking, ending with sleeping, making time for meals and other activities at certain times. There is a rhythm to your week with specific time to work, time to socialize. Sunday may be a day of worship or a day to prepare for the rest of the week. There is a rhythm to your month as well. There is a specific time of month that you pay your mortgage or rent, along with the rest of your bills. If you're a woman, you notice monthly physical changes. The moon will light up the sky for us each month. Every few months there is a rhythmical change in the earth's energy that represents the life cycle, from the loss of deciduous tree leaves in the fall, to the pausing chill and hibernation of winter, to the rebirth of wildflowers and blossoms in the spring, and back to a warm pause in the summer heat. You will experience variations from the extremes of each seasonal cycle, but it will cycle nonetheless.

With the many changes we continuously face, it's necessary to have stability in our lives. The Earth, in relation to the Moon and Sun, creates this stability, this rhythm for us to settle into and to move with. Although we witness dependable seasons, we also witness weather extremes within the stability. Notice how grateful you feel when the seasons change. You return to a known energy, and although each season is new again, it is just a continuation of the pattern. If you haven't experienced weather extremes, you can notice on the news how grateful people are to get back to "normal," once a weather tragedy passes.

This is just Mother Nature communicating to us, just as our body does when it gets sick. We can interpret the message in any number of ways. "Be grateful for what you have" is what I always hear. It is what I have learned to hear, anyway. At this point of my life I am aware that I certainly can choose to hear something else, but do not see the value in that. Will it, for example, serve me to believe that the things that interrupt my rhythm are designed to hurt me? This would be the opposite of gratitude and is a choice. If I'm blaming things in my life for my pain, I am not in gratitude and also forfeiting my responsibility in creating my life to my liking.

An important note to share here is that this book was written for the purpose of life healing—in this very moment as well as all future ones. We all have many, many experiences, both of extreme joy and of tragedy. This book neither addresses extreme tragedies nor tries to make light of them. In applying the exercises, I do realize that there are certain challenges like the loss of a child or a parent or any loved one that turns your world inside out. These exercises will not touch the depth of sorrow in these situations. Please apply these tools to everyday life, that has ups and downs with jobs and relationships, et cetera, but if grieving is necessary—deep, heart-wrenching grieving—these exercises will be untouchable, and this I understand and expect.

On the other hand I see much drama in our lives over little things that appear to the person to need grieving that are really quite superficial and theatrical. Often times we realize this only after the situation has passed. As you learn to live from the perspective of gratitude you will begin to observe the many tiny annoyances that get way too much attention, negative attention.

Gratitude is a belief system. This is why I put this chapter under the Spirit section. It's a belief system available for you to choose to embrace. I believe that all things that happen in our lives are purposely designed for our personal growth experiences. Each challenge offers us specific opportunities to practice love. The path to love is gratitude.

So, if each challenge is an opportunity and nothing happens by accident, why not surrender to it? "All is as it should be," therefore, summarizes the entire practice. And practice it is. The practice requires awareness and choice—the same thing over and over. Practicing gratitude is living in love—love of *everything* in your life! If you need to shift in what you are doing so that you can be grateful, do so. Gratitude is a belief and it is an action.

> ***And the circle is complete.***
>
> Gratitude is an action that stimulates more action.
>
> Actions based in gratitude feed the belief that all is as it should be.

Some of you may have trouble with the statement "All is as it should be." As you examine your world you may think that our government is not as it should be, or that starving children are not "as it should be," or the loss of your job is not "as it should be." Perhaps these life experiences are not as you would like them to be, but they are anyway. This shows us how much control we have over our world—not much. And since we do not have control, we can focus on what we do have—and that's influence. If you want to direct your life through beautiful experiences, you will want to influence your world through love, right? You wouldn't create beautiful experiences through anger or resentment or sadness, right? In the moment, it may feel like you can because your energy is strong and focused, but if you step out of the heated moment you realize that although the situation may not be what you want, the negative emotions do not help the situation at large.

Once we realize that certain situations will be, regardless of if we want them or not, and that we can't "control" any outcomes, we begin to see that it is unnecessary to be in an emotion that doesn't support movement in any way. Being sad keeps things stuck. Being angry has movement to it, it's not stuck like sadness, but in what direction are you moving with anger? Although sadness and anger are natural and normal emotions, it isn't helpful to stay stuck in them. The best way to move out of your stuck emotion and to begin creating things in your life that you desire is to focus on your intent. If your intent is to have a full and beautiful life, you'll need to influence your world through actions of love. Your influence through anger will not create a beautiful life. I am speaking very generally but this is how you begin to understand it. Feel the words you are reading and surrender to the power of the truth of them. In summary, put your energy where you want it. Align your energy with the type of energy you want to create in your life. A great way to practice this is to notice gratitude of all things that you have now. Sure, there are probably things in your life that you do not want; just let them be and give your attention rather to those things that you do love.

Perhaps right now you are sad or angry about something, and these words are just hogwash to you. Recognize your sadness or anger. Choose to stay there as long as you want. Once you're ready, you can choose to feel the emotion of gratitude. For what, you ask? For getting through the experience, for having all of the other wonderful things in your life that you're forgetting about in this moment, for the life you are now creating from a feeling that feels good, for noticing you just needed a little downtime, or for needing to take a run to release energy—for whatever you can find that is good about your life.

As you focus with gratitude on what you do have, the things you don't have will dwindle out of your consciousness and the things that you do have will be magnified. By focusing on what you do have, you will create more of the same. By living in gratitude, you remind yourself over and over about what you do have. You cannot have more than one thought at a time. Your option is to choose to focus on what you love, what you are grateful for. The little gratitudes will fuel bigger and bigger ones. If you really would like to master this practice, you can study the work of Abraham Hicks through the book *Ask and It Is Given* by Esther and Jerry Hicks.

Now you are participating as actively as you can in your life. You are creating your experiences, which create your health. What an awesome opportunity to live and to share!

The Gratitude Journal

Each night before you go to bed, close your day with gratitude.

Think back to the first event of your day today. Write down a simple gratitude for waking to a new day.

Continue writing a gratitude for each event that occurred during this day.

Don't skip any event. Find a way to be grateful for *everything*, especially the difficult experiences.

Lastly, close with a gratitude before closing your eyes and resting peacefully all night long, ready to wake to a new day.

This exercise allows you to put closure on every day.
It allows your spirit a safe and comfortable place
to rest along with your body and your mind . . .
It gives you a chance to wake refreshed
with all of your resources available.

∞ Chapter 23 ∞

The Spirit

∫

Forgiveness

Forgiveness is the result of gratitude. It is not an action. It is not something you need to do. It happens when you are in gratitude. If you are in a state of gratitude for everything in your life, you are not holding anyone or anything hostage. By freeing yourself of anger or hatred, you have also freed others.

Most of my patients, though, find it easier to do things for themselves if they believe they are doing it for others. For example, "I'm pregnant and so I will eat very healthily for the benefit of my baby." Or, "My husband is tired of my PMS so I thought I'd do something about it." Or, "My wife wants me to quit smoking, so here I am." So often, I am treating a husband or a child because their wife or mother wanted them to come in for a visit. I have found it to be so important that the individual who is in my patient's chair chose for herself to come in for healing. This is the only time that true healing has a chance.

One by one, as each of us does his or her own work, the planet at large begins to shift. As a whole we are all moving together, towards something. We all play a very big part in the direction that the energy of the Earth is heading. If we want to live forever and get the most out of all of the progress we are making as an advancing society, we've got to first start with gratitude. This is the thread to success. If we do not create out of gratitude, we will face our destruction. If we do not consciously choose gratitude, we are simply living by default. Gratitude is the action necessary for a fulfilling lifetime experience and expresses itself very clearly in our health and our personal worlds that we create.

Any negative thought you have accelerates destruction. Any positive thought you have facilitates creation. Stop and examine your life to see if there is anyone that you hold any bit of resentment, anger, frustration, jealousy or bitterness towards. Notice who is experiencing these emotions. You are. The person delivering the energy that creates these emotions inside of you may very well be feeling the same thing—big deal. Your life is about you. You create your reactions. You own your emotions. We can't blame it on anyone else. Reflect back to the very last exercise and notice that you have the potential to be grateful for that person in spite of the pain you previously attached to that person. Choosing gratitude allows forgiveness and you will become free. As your healing path unfolds, you will see that the only person requiring forgiveness is you.

I understand that you may still believe that it's important to forgive someone for their wrongdoing that affected you. Why do you believe that you owe them any favor? You do, however, certainly deserve to forgive yourself for allowing these thoughts. This is done simply by finding a way to be grateful for this funny world that we live in.

My proposal to you is to join the path of healing. This will not only significantly impact you, but it will also affect your intimate world, and even the world you don't feel you've ever met.

∞ Chapter 24 ∞

Spirit

$$\int$$

Love

This whole book has been about nothing but love. The first step in healing of any manner is self-observation—becoming more conscious of the self. You may desire healing in a relationship, or of an illness, or of a financial situation. Once you become centered in self-observation, you will be able to recognize and embrace experiences that create and reflect self-honor. You constantly get feedback about whether or not your choices are seated in self-honor. If your internal health is harmonious, peaceful and joyful, then you are creating through self-honor. If your external world is harmonious, peaceful and joyful, then you are creating through self-honor. The more you practice self-observation, the more readily you will recognize when you are not in self-honor. That is how specific your feedback is. Your body and your world will get your attention when you are not in self-love. By automatically recognizing the lack of ease in your physical body or your physical world, you are reconnected to the practice of love. The more consistently you practice this, the less you will be influenced by chaos and stress. You simply will not create it. The creation of your outer world is an absolute reflection of your inner world. As you become more centered in self-love, you will naturally begin attracting people to you who reserve energy for your highest good and vice versa. You will know immediately if a particular experience is the correct one for you. This applies to employers and employees, to real estate agents, to friends, to doctors, and even to places you frequent for shopping and socializing. Self-love creates the stage of your world.

The road that maintains the practice in love is gratitude. Whenever your attention is drawn to knowing that, in that moment, you are not in self-honor, choose to be grateful instead—for something. This is where I find patients need most assistance. As you understand the ground rules and practice them it will get easier and more and more fun. Be gentle with yourself. Understanding the practice is the first step. This is the intellectual step. Bridging your understanding of the rules to the emotional owning of them is what takes the most amount of time and energy. As you become more harmonious in self-love, there will be no other way in which you could treat others. You would simply know of no other way. This would be your dance—circular, like the seasons, constantly feeding more and more of the harmony within you. If your daily practice maintains itself in a forward direction, it is a circle. If you slow down, get bored, or get scared, the circle becomes choppy. It is your dance; create it from what feels best.

In our full lives we participate in a dance with each other. At times the dance is lovely and graceful and absolutely beautiful. At other times it appears that we never took a lesson! Regardless of who we are dancing with, the lesson is always about learning how to choose love.

With the pure practice of love, all *else* dissolves. As everything but love dissolves, all is well. The affirmation "all is as it should be" allows you the privilege of *living* "all is well"—not just liking and understanding the words. If you allow your intellect to know that all is as it should be and your emotional being becomes this, the fuel and thriving circle is maintained.

Since I was born with an incredible fascination with the human experience, I know for certain that I will forever be delighted to continue learning the magic of simple philosophies and seeing the benefits manifest as health in the physical expression of the body. I know that I will never cease being amazed at the absolute perfection of each and every experience. I am amazed at the simplicity, yet complexity, of the anatomy of the human body and its interplay with the non-physical body. There isn't one thing in our life that doesn't contribute to every reaction. There are no accidents. You've probably read in the works of many masters that this is truth. I know this by feeling it and by witnessing this truth manifesting itself in my patients' health or lack of it. Like you, I get tired of practice—eating well, exercising routinely, not permitting stress to affect my sleep, being the right person to my family, friends, and patients. It does get hard—excuse me, more challenging. It's not hard, it's simple. Well, I'm human, just like all of you. I'm addicted to figuring out how to maintain that delicate respect for all of me. We are all complex. The only simple solution to "figuring it all out" is to remain in a state of joy regardless of what is occurring in our lives, to recognize when we aren't feeling good about something, to change what we are doing or thinking, and to maintain the highest level of respect for absolutely all of life. This is the practice. This is the magic.

There will forever be at least two sides to every idea. There is absolutely—never—only one way. Love, however, is the only successful path to whichever side your viewpoint or perception is stemming from. It is the answer to every question ever asked. It is time to open our hearts and allow all things to happen.

∞ Chapter 25 ∞

Healing Paths

∫

Same Condition, Different Journey

I'd like to present to you how two different people healed from the same condition in entirely different ways. Both patients suffered from rheumatoid arthritis. Both were females, both were middle-aged, and both lived in the same area.

The first story is about Lynda (*I have changed the names in these stories*). She had suffered from arthritis for more than twenty years and had gone through all of the conventional treatments including pain and anti-inflammatory medications, oral and injectable steroids, and even gold injections. She sat in my office, obviously deformed by the illness, complaining of chronic pain with certain times of exacerbation, without any experience of remission. I went through her history and noticed that her symptoms started when she was in her late twenties at a time when her health otherwise was unremarkable. She didn't have any surgeries and was on medication for her arthritis symptoms as well as for daily migraines and birth control pills as her contraceptive choice. One of her aunts had arthritis as well.

Her laboratory workup showed high triglycerides with normal liver enzymes, thyroid function, kidney function, and immune function. Her sedimentation rate was high as well, which is a non-specific marker of inflammation.

In evaluating lifestyle I question patients about diet, elimination patterns, exercise, sleep patterns, stress level and the management of it. Her nutrition was common with bagels and cream cheese for breakfast, hamburger or salad for lunch and some sort of protein for dinner with pasta or a potato or rice. She drank little water, one glass of wine each evening with dinner and a Diet Coke with lunch and dinner. Moreover, Lynda loved sweets. She couldn't exercise because of the pain. She tended to be constipated, having bowel movements every two to three days. Her sleep was poor, she was waking frequently with difficulty getting back to sleep and she was considering taking a sleeping pill. Lynda's stress level wasn't particularly high outside of her low level of wellness.

Arthritis symbolically reflects a convenient way that the body stores waste. By reviewing her lifestyle I saw many waste-accumulating possibilities which I will list:

- Bagels and cream cheese—wheat and dairy are commonly difficult foods for the body to digest efficiently and are considered for most people to be inflammatory foods. Since she has an inflammatory condition, I would suspect that these foods are not helping her health.

- Wheat again at lunch in the bun of the burger along with arachidonic acid in meat that is also pro-inflammatory. Not all people need to avoid meat and wheat, but until we identify what is contributing to her inflammation, meat will be suspected.

- Water is cleansing to the body and assists in carrying waste away from cells and to the digestive tract. Lynda's water intake is low.

- Wine challenges liver metabolism by congesting the detoxification pathways. As the liver's job of detoxification is compromised by the daily use of wine, there will be more systemic inflammation.

- Diet Coke contains artificial chemicals and caffeine that challenge detoxification. Caffeine is similar to adrenalin biochemically and will inadvertently affect the function of our adrenal glands. Our adrenal glands create our circadian rhythm which is our wake and sleep cycle. Furthermore, the adrenal glands secrete our anti-inflammatory hormones. Since caffeine impacts her adrenal glands directly, she will have more inflammation.

- All of her medications are processed through the liver, challenging and congesting the liver which further compromises her ability to naturally detoxify.
- She is inactive, rendering her cells idle, down-regulating cellular metabolism, which impacts both cellular assimilation of nutrition and waste removal.
- Lynda's sleep is compromised. The only reason the body needs sleep is to restore itself. During sleep the body enters the state of anabolism, or building. This is the only time the body does this. Inappropriate rest prevents the body from rebuilding and instead it stays in a constant state of degeneration.

The most obvious treatment for this patient was to detoxify her body. I chose not to initially run food allergy or nutrient testing on her as her toxicity was so obvious. I first wanted the opportunity to clean up the muddy water in this patient and do further testing later on if necessary.

It is possible to detoxify gently or aggressively. I usually describe both methods to my patients and have them decide which will work best with their lifestyle. The gentle detoxification is done by limiting the diet to foods that are considered to be non-inflammatory. Aggressive detoxification is done by replacing all food with detoxification drinks to be used throughout the day, which contain nutrients that enhance detoxification.

Lynda decided to be aggressive. I designed a detoxification plan specifically for her and asked her to call me when all of her pain was gone. I encouraged her to journal her experience because the physical waste layers she was going to shed held emotional layers that also got laid down in the physical layers. It is impossible to cleanse just the physical body. Remember how intertwined and complex and extraordinary the human experience is. An aggressive detoxification will stir the whole pot!

I inquired if Lynda would consider an alternative method of birth control, the diaphragm, which is a barrier method that does not manipulate her hormones nor challenge the liver unnecessarily. She was willing to do so.

Ten days later, Lynda called the office to let me know that her pain was only about 80% gone but that she was missing food. Otherwise she had no complaints. Her energy was improving, her focus at work was improving, her sleep was significantly better and she had not taken migraine medication in six days. She was pleased with her progress but very much wanting to eat.

Since her momentum was now going in the right direction, I felt very comfortable altering her plan because if the change in her plan interrupted the momentum we would know immediately that it was the wrong choice. Together we chose to bring in cooked vegetables only for a few days and then to bring in proteins like fish and chicken along with salads. She was more than happy with the change.

We followed up six weeks later. She hadn't taken a pain pill for arthritis in three weeks. She did have stiffness, but no actual pain. At this point I asked her to supplement her diet with fish oil capsules and digestive enzymes and to introduce food slowly, noticing if any one food exacerbated her condition.

Three months later she had a clear list of foods that if she stayed away from, would keep her symptom free. She didn't mind the diet very much as her freedom from pain was worth the restrictions.

As time goes on, the restrictions may become more difficult. If so, she has the option to continue in the same manner with her diet, and adjust her view of health. She can be guided to realize that the foods she had to avoid gave her freedom. This viewpoint, if mastered redefines the foods she had to avoid from 'restrictions' to 'freedom.' In this case she is choosing, hopefully effortlessly so, to redefine her world from the perspective of wellness with a viewpoint of freedom rather than from a perspective of illness with a viewpoint of victim. For some this is easy. For others this is a tremendous struggle. Neither is right or wrong, it just directs the individual journey. For the first time in Lynda's life she was feeling freedom and was exhilarated to not need to define herself as a victim any longer. She was complete.

For those to whom this does not come so easily, it is important to continue the journey a little longer. At this fork in the road I personally explore a homeopathic remedy which, if the right one is identified, can offer the patient more freedom, by eliminating her impaired ability to ingest the food without causing inflammation when exposed to the food. With a cleaner body, a homeopathic remedy has great potential and it will be easier to identify a remedy. For simplicity's sake in this book, homeopathic remedies are vibrational remedies. There is no identifiable substance in the remedy; rather, it contains the energy that matches the individual's energy to balance the complete system. And, in addition, I offer Mental-Emotional Reprogramming sessions to those who struggle more with the physical choices they are making. You will learn more of this with the next patient's story.

The second story is about Suzanne. She came to me for the treatment of rheumatoid arthritis, with symptoms of constantly stiff, painful hands, which impaired her functioning so significantly that she was unable to cook for her family anymore. She did have pain in other joints but the pain was predominantly in her hands. She was taking pain medicine consistently, and still the pain never went away completely. She described the pain as coming on rather quickly about one year ago. Otherwise she was in pretty good health, with some complaints of fatigue and sleeplessness.

Her knuckles were enlarged with some distortion in her wrists and she showed me that her hand strength was notably weak. When I asked Suzanne about the stress in her life she shared that about six months ago her husband died in a car accident. The accident actually occurred a year ago with the last six months of his life being on life support in the facility. She has gone through grief counseling and is currently living a life with her three sons at home.

It is not customary for me to offer emotional work on my first visit. The emotional work I do is a specific technique that I call Mental-Emotional Reprogramming. I begin with a meditation to help the patient bring her awareness and focus into the self, and then connect her with the memory of the onset of the condition. When a person plays a video in their mind about the event or condition needing healing, the physical body inevitably will have a response or reaction to the images. Since Suzanne's symptoms began at the onset of losing her husband, I thought there was enough of a correlation between her arthritis and her life situation that we should start there.

My focus in evaluating patients is to identify a link between the onset of symptoms and a life situation—be it a diet change, a relationship change, a move, anything that has a time concurrence. It shows me what energy is affecting the system most aggressively. It may be an emotion, a nutrient, a stressful situation, a drug, a surgery, a loss, a financial shift—whatever the event, the energy of the event guides the therapeutic plan. It is not essential to have a specific association, but it is very helpful.

On this particular visit, I bypassed the physical exam and laboratory testing. Suzanne was more than happy to look at the correlation between her husband's loss and her symptoms, as she had never considered this before.

We began the Mental-Emotional Reprogramming process. After she was relaxed in her body, and her mind became still and focused inward, I began the process of her remembering. First I had her play a video in her mind of the time prior to her husband's accident. With as much detail as possible I had her watch a video of when her husband was alive and they were sharing their life. Then I had her move forward with the video to the day that she got news of the accident, and to remember as much detail as possible about where she was when she got the call—as many details as she could remember. After a few moments I asked her to stop watching the video and to bring her awareness into her physical body and to notice what her body felt like. She immediately said that her hands were balled into tight fists. I saw the fists she was making also and they looked a lot more energetic than the strength she demonstrated to me earlier. She said her body felt tense all over. Since her fists got her attention first, I guided her to keep her attention there and to just communicate one thing silently to them. I asked her to silently thank her hands for getting her attention. I did not want her to be grateful for the tension, the tightness, just for the guidance of her physical body as it responded to the video in her mind. The very moment she started the silent process of gratitude to her hands she started sobbing—uncontrollably. She wanted to stop the work, sat up, grabbed several tissues and sobbed for what seemed to be about twenty minutes.

    She reached out for my hands and looked into my eyes and said, "I wanted to hold onto Jack for dear life! My hands got stuck desperately clinging to him!" Her sobbing continued.

    I waited until she was ready to speak. She stood to throw out the tissues. She sat down and opened her hands gently on her legs, staring at them. She softly looked up and said, "This is the first time I don't have any pain in my hands whatsoever. I didn't take pain medication this morning because I wasn't sure what you would want to see, and I am, in this moment, pain free."

For Suzanne, the most important part of healing was to be able to release the cramped emotion of terror and grief of losing her husband from living in the body. This is an excellent example of just how energetic our bodies are. This had nothing to do with nutrition or medication or supplementation. This was about how her energy got stuck, her vibration that matched health shifted because of a shocking emotion. Emotions affect our vibration just as strongly as food, as strongly as medications. In this particular case, it was the cause of her illness.

These very different stories demonstrate how the diagnosis isn't the appropriate place to start if our choice is to heal. The diagnosis tells the end of the story. The end of a story does not summarize any book; it is the endpoint, it is the result of the story. The story is what deserves the attention if we are to heal.

If prevention is the goal, if decreasing acute outcomes of a chronic disease is the goal, if treatment of chronic conditions is the goal, conventional medicine is not the place to go to get answers. This is the territory of the field of Naturopathic Medicine. Although Naturopathic Medicine is alive and thriving and saturated with patients in Arizona where I live and practice, it is my heart's desire to see this countrywide—worldwide. The planet depends on it.

∞ Chapter 26 ∞

Healing Paths

∫

The Real Deal

And so, with great emotion, I complete this book with tremendous hopes to uplift you as you choose healing. May you seek the limitless potential within you that has not yet been tapped. This book has been written for all people.

I believe it to be imperative that more and more people realize how important it is to invest in our own well-being. The mere truth that our inner health is a mirror of our world and vice versa needs first to be understood, then valued, then invested in.

It is simply impossible to be a peaceful, harmonious and balanced individual inside, and create a personal world of chaos with unhealthy relationships, lack of financial achievement, and unruly children. It's not a fit; it goes against nature. At the same time it is impossible to experience a chaotic internal experience with symptoms that distract you from optimal well-being, while creating an effortless life with optimal relationships, wealth and children. Healing your body heals your personal world.

I'd like to give you a flavor of the real deal as it relates to my life. I practice all of the exercises that I have provided for you. I practice. I get frustrated when I don't remember to practice. I enter periods of eternal gratitude that seem as though they can never be interrupted—but then I get a chance to practice again. This is life.

We are all perfect. Practice means perfection. If we are practicing to be the best we can be, we will be the best we can be, and we are perfect. Does this mean that I never have a bad day or a bad experience or always have the immediate tools at hand to handle a challenging situation in the moment? Of course not. I am human. You are human.

Have fun with your challenges, rejoice in your successes and try to always choose things that make you happy. Nobody outside of you can choose your personal happiness unless you allow them to. People do have the right to judge you, but who cares? You know by now that their judgment is a reflection of their own insecurity and has nothing to do with you. Sounds easier than it is? Not if you keep practicing.

With every thought your biochemistry is being created. Every choice that you make in creating your life is born out of an emotion. Your emotions and thoughts are interwoven into any design you choose. Your physical health is intimately supported within this web. Be the web!

My practice has such varying types of patients, with limitless types of personalities, and a multitude of different expectations. This is the fun part as a physician. The varying complexities of each patient and condition are both beautiful and challenging at the same time. My trust in the healing process is the very thing that keeps my job simple. It may be magical and it may be miraculous but it is always real. The fuel that keeps me going is the healing that I am privileged to witness daily.

The big picture, the images and feelings that come to you from reading this book, is where we as a society have evolved to today, and it not only deserves our focus and attention, but it is also absolutely essential that we open our hearts to it. For evolution to unfold with beauty and grace, we, individually and together, must unite from our higher perspective. It is the real deal. The more of us that are committed to healing, the greater the experience of this world. This is my prayer.

Naturopathic Organizations

The American Association of Naturopathic Physicians (AANP)
3201 New Mexico Avenue, NW Suite 350
Washington, DC 20016
Phone: 866.538.2267
Fax: 202.274.1992
Website: www.naturopathic.org

The AANP is the national professional society representing naturopathic physicians who are licensed or eligible for licensing as primary care providers.

There are individual state naturopathic associations, each providing a representative to the House of Delegates to establish policies for the AANP.

Naturopathic Medical Schools

Bastyr University
14500 Juanita Dr. NE
Kenmore, Washington 98028-4966
Phone: 425.823.1300
Fax: 425.823.6222
Website: www.bastyr.edu

Boucher Institute of Naturopathic Medicine
#200—558 Carnarvon St.
New Westminster, British Columbia V3M 5Y6 Canada
Phone: 604.777.9981
Fax: 604.777.9982
Website: www.binm.org

Canadian College of Naturopathic Medicine
1255 Sheppard Ave. East
Toronto, Ontario, M2K 1E2 Canada
Phone: 416.498.1576
Toll-Free: 866.241.2266
Website: www.ccnm.edu

National College of Naturopathic Medicine
049 SW Porter Street
Portland, Oregon 97201
Phone: 503.552.1555
Fax: 503.499.0022
Website: www.ncmn.edu

Southwest College of Naturopathic Medicine
2140 E. Broadway Road
Tempe, Arizona 85282
Phone: 480.858.9100
Fax: 480.858.9116
Website: www.scnm.edu

University of Bridgeport College of Naturopathic Medicine
60 Lafayette St.
Bridgeport, Connecticut 06601-2449
Phone: 203.576.4109
Website: www.bridgeport.edu

Commonly Asked Questions

What is an NMD?
A Naturopathic Medical Doctor.

What is the difference between an NMD and an MD?
Licensing titles are determined by licensing boards. The Naturopathic Board of Medical Examiners offers the medical board exams and licenses NMDs. The different board exams reflect the educational background of the candidate as well as physician privileges.

What is the educational background of an NMD?
Medical school is similar to conventional medical school, consisting of the advanced sciences, clinical and physical diagnosis, pathology, minor surgery and pharmacology. In addition, naturopathic students study nutrition, homeopathy, botanical medicine, acupuncture and Chinese medicine, natural childbirth, and physical medicine, which includes spinal manipulation and hydrotherapy. Premed schooling is a requirement prior to entering naturopathic medical school similar to conventional medical school. Postgraduate internships are not a requirement for NMD's, but are available and advisable. Currently,

internship hours are blended into the educational training prior to sitting for the board exams.

Information in the table below was derived from the AANP and compares hours of study between naturopathic medical schools and conventional medical schools. The average of the Naturopathic Medical Schools is derived from the following schools: National College of Naturopathic Medicine, Bastyr University and Southwest College of Naturopathic Medicine. The average of the Conventional Medical Schools is derived from the following schools: Johns Hopkins, Yale, and Stanford University.

	Naturopathic Medial Colleges	Conventional Medical Colleges
Basic and Clinical Sciences	1535	1524
Clinical Diagnosis	1664	3393
Nutrition	135	0
Naturopathic therapeutics	707	0

What do you do as an NMD?
I am a family practitioner. I treat all people. Since I practice naturopathic medicine, my approach is different than what you would expect at a typical conventional doctor's office. I don't treat the condition as much as I treat the person who has the condition.

What is naturopathic medicine?
A system of primary health care whereby the licensed practitioner diagnoses and treats the person based on the cause of the illness. It is based on the premise that our DNA expresses itself uniquely based on exposures,

deficiencies, excesses, trauma, grief, stress, addictions, etc. Due to the many factors that influence our health, Naturopathic Physicians treat the person who has the condition, rather than the condition itself. The condition, however, is interesting as it helps us understand where physiology became interrupted, causing lack of harmony in a particular person.

What would your approach be to a new patient coming into your office?
The initial private consultation lasts about one hour. The first thing I look at is the reason they came in. Next, I briefly scan over their known family history. I explore how long they've suffered to see if there is an identifiable life event that may have predisposed or launched their condition. In addition, I need to know what the life of this person has been like as far as major stressors, dietary practices, sleep patterns, medication and supplement exposures and surgeries. There is a lot of exploring in the first visit. If time permits, a physical exam is done either at this visit or at the following one. Laboratory testing is prescribed if necessary to gain more information. The initial treatment plan is specific to each person.

I'm used to a ten-minute doctor visit. Is an hour really necessary?
Pathology doesn't just appear one day. Pathology is the end point. Pathology is physiology gone wrong. It's

easy to take a medication to suppress a symptom. It's quick to cut out an irregular cell. The first hour consult is a mere reflection of the essence of time that goes into healing. It took you a while to get sick. Expect to take some time to get well.

Does insurance cover NMDs?
Rarely does insurance cover my services; however, almost all insurance will cover my prescriptions for medications and radiology studies.

Do you take insurance at your office?
No. Your insurance may cover my services. We, however, do not bill insurance from our office. If your insurance will cover my services, you can submit your bill that you paid to us and have your insurance company reimburse you. We provide the codes that your insurance company will need to process the claim.

Do you prescribe medications?
I do prescribe medications when necessary and have respect for this privilege.

Do you prescribe hormones for menopause? There seems to be so much controversy over this issue.
I do prescribe dio-identical hormone replacement therapy if needed. Menopausal transition is a very personal decision. I respect individual choices as long as they do not increase risks and are not made out of fear.

Do you do laboratory testing?
I prescribe laboratory testing as well as imaging studies like X-rays, ultrasounds, CTs and MRIs when necessary.

Could you be my primary care physician?
I can be your primary care physician. Some patients use me in this role and come to me for both acute and chronic complaints. Some patients keep a primary care physician from their insurance plan for acute conditions and use my services more for their chronic complaints.

If I needed to go to the hospital, would you treat me there?
I do not have hospital privileges. Some NMDs have become hospitalists. I prefer to not obtain these privileges. Personally, if I were in the hospital, I would want to be under the care of someone who is trained to function best in the urgent setting. I would want the best for my patients also and know that it wouldn't be me in this situation.

If you are my primary care doctor and I have to go to the hospital, what happens?
If you needed to go to the hospital, you would enter through the emergency room. If you got admitted, the hospital would assign you a physician to oversee your care.

Would you consult with my primary care doctor if necessary?
Yes, absolutely.

Do you practice anti-aging medicine?
I don't like to use the word "anti" in a treatment protocol unless you are in a life threatening situation or if your quality of life is significantly affected. I do prescribe quality of life enhancement therapies, especially in healthy individuals who want to age gracefully.

Is it common for someone to go to a Naturopathic Physician?
With each passing year, graduates from the Naturopathic Medical Schools are starting up new practices in our country. Even still, only eleven states have legalized Naturopathic Physicians. In time it is my hope that each of the 50 states will legalize the practice of Naturopathic Medicine. Due to this dilemma, I, like other NMDs, do have patients from around the country and the world. The process of legalization is slow.

What is the difference between an N.M.D. and an N.D.?
The title is dictated by the state in which a physician is licensed. The state board exams are independent of other states. The states that do not license for pharmacy or surgery privileges designate the title N.D. In states where

pharmacy and surgery privileges exist, the designated title can be N.D. or N.M.D.

Which States have currently legalized Naturopathic Medicine?

Alaska
Arizona
California
Connecticut
District of Columbia
Hawaii
Kansas
Maine
Montana
New Hampshire
Oregon
Utah
Vermont
Washington
US Territories: Puerto Rico and Virgin Islands